REGENERATIVE MEDICINE

Proven Ways to Eliminate Pain, Restore Mobility, and Repair Athletic Injuries

DR. DARLA L. LOGAN, NMD, MBA

Published by Best Seller Publishing®, Pasadena, CA
Best Seller Publishing® is a registered trademark
Printed in the United States of America.
ISBN 978-1-946978-12-7

For more information, please write:
Best Seller Publishing®
1346 Walnut Street, #205
Pasadena, CA 91106
or call 1(626) 765 9750
Toll Free: 1(844) 850-3500
Visit us online at: www.BestSellerPublishing.org

To my patients past, present,
and future.

Table of Contents

Acknowledgement

This work would not have been possible without the mentorship and friendship of Dr. Mark Rudderham, NMD. You took me from student to physician. The impact you have had on my life is far too great to express adequately on paper. You are one of the most brilliant physicians I have encountered, a "lumberjack," "mad scientist," loving father, and devoted husband. You promised me on my first day that you would teach me not only the science but also the art of medicine. You prepared me, encouraged me, and entertained me. I am forever grateful that our paths crossed.

INTRODUCTION

Pain: The Great Motivator

There are few weeks that go by that I don't get the opportunity to answer the question, "What made you choose medicine?" or "Can you tell me about yourself as a healer?" The truth is, I don't refer to myself as a healer; the term just doesn't resonate with me. Let me explain why. When I think of the term *healer*, I conjure up all sorts of images in my mind, none of which I equate with myself, my skills, or my knowledge. I, as a person, can do absolutely nothing to heal another person's pain or illness. So for me, the term *healer* gives me credit for something I can never accomplish. I consider myself more of a facilitator. What I can do is facilitate healing—give information, treatments, medication, or supplements that allow healing to take place. The real work is done by the person following my direction and his or her body.

Having said that, I got into medicine for the purpose of having a career that would allow me to be the person I wanted to be, to affect the world in a meaningful way on an individual level. As I went through the process of figuring out who I wanted to be in the world, one thing stood out: I wanted to be able to give people options to live a life that was meaningful to them. And as a doctor, this is what I do every day. I work with people to solve problems that are preventing them from having a fulfilling, quality life. This happens on many levels. However, pain is a niche area in my practice. Pain motivates people to take action. Think about knee pain, back pain, headaches, or shoulder pain. These conditions can be quite debilitating. While pain in general has many causes, physical injury and disease are among the most common reasons for pain.

Conventionally, there are limited options for treatment: pain medication, both over the counter and prescription; physical therapy; and surgery. In my experience, there can be significant limitations to the effectiveness of each of those options. Many people have gone so far as to have surgery, resulting in either temporary or no relief. So when you have tried everything your doctor has to offer and still haven't been able to get relief, where to do you go? What do you try? It's frustrating, limiting, and quite disempowering.

What if we take a different approach to pain? What if we are willing to toss out some of the conventional thinking and go back to the drawing board? What if we take what we know and expand the way we use that knowledge? What if we give the body what it needs to do the thing it does best—heal? What if we are willing to get out of the way? What kind of results are we likely to have? These are the questions that flood my mind daily. It's this type of thinking that led me to regenerative medicine, and I am excited to discuss these pain management options with you.

Physical pain is something I have lived with, endured, and survived. It changed my life and made me a person I never thought I would become: cranky and impatient. At times, I thought death would be easier than the life I had because that life was punctuated with pain. Every morning, the alarm would sound, and the cycle would begin again. The first thing I would do was an evaluation of my body—how severe my aches were that morning and what areas of my body they affected. Then I would do an assessment of what was on my agenda that day—the meetings I had and the people I needed to interact with. It wasn't but a short time later when I would reach for the pain medication.

I was fortunate as I never fell into the trap of narcotic pain medication, but I was popping ibuprofen like it was candy. It was very common for me to take 800 milligrams of ibuprofen every two hours. Even though I was exceeding the maximum dose on most days, the pain wasn't gone; it was just blunted—barely bearable. Looking back, I realize that my expectation wasn't even to be rid of the pain; it was just to have a manageable pain. I'm not sure I thought I ever would be free of pain. I just wanted to be able to get through the day.

I remember thinking to myself, "I am far too young to feel this old." My life was filled with a series of things I had to endure rather than enjoyment, and each day became a countdown. I was counting down the hours until the workday was over and I could lie on the couch where I at least could be still and quiet, and no one would require anything of me. I was counting down the hours until I could allow the tears to run down my face without a feeling of reprisal. I was miserable. I suspect many can relate to how I was feeling at the time.

It was a strange feeling when I became pain-free. I didn't even notice that the pain was gone until it returned. Then I couldn't believe the excruciating level of pain I had endured for so long and how much my body had suffered. Honestly, it was quite shocking.

Pain has been a part of my life for as long as I can remember. I didn't always have pain in my body, but that didn't stop the pain from being a huge component of my life. As a child, I was affected by my mother's pain. Back in my earliest memories, there was hardly a day that went by that I didn't watch my mother suffer. Even the most mundane acts caused her to wince. If she sat too long, if she walked too far, if she stood too long—activities that many of us take for granted—she would be in pain.

Lumbar scoliosis was the official diagnosis, compounded by a neck fracture and natural vertebral fusion of her cervical vertebrae, following a fall down the stairs at age 10. I remember her trips to the doctor and hearing reports that she would need a wheelchair and that the only thing that would allow her to continue walking was a metal rod placed in her spine. Surgery and pain pills—two things my mother was dead set against—were the options presented to her. We often went to the family chiropractor, and he was instrumental in keeping my mother walking, but he couldn't manage her pain well. Every movement and every step of every day caused her excruciating pain, but she pressed through it.

I also remember a time when my mother was active. I remember her playing softball and working very physically demanding jobs to help provide for our family. I remember her building frames to pour sidewalks in our yard. Pretty much anything she wanted to do, she did. But as the years went by, things changed. Her pain became increasingly worse, and she seemed to age quickly.

By the time she was in her early 30s, she no longer played sports, and although she still had a physically demanding job, that was about all she could do. At the end of the day, she ached, but she ached at the beginning of the day as well. I could never tell if the pain was worse in the morning or at night because it seemed like it just never went away.

Don't get me wrong; I never felt as though I missed out on anything in my childhood. My mother was always present, but I noticed as I got older and, subsequently, as she got older, that there were fewer and fewer things she participated in. I remember her sitting on the sidelines when we went ice-skating in Central Park with my nieces, and I remember her hiding behind a curtain so that she could avoid dancing at my brother's wedding. These activities were just too painful for her.

I think most people didn't realize how much she was suffering. She looked healthy. Therefore, she had to be healthy. In actuality, she was probably more stubborn than healthy. She was too stubborn to stop, give up, and resign herself to the wheelchair she had been sentenced to years earlier. Her quality of life was certainly affected, and her options for regaining a life without pain were not really options and still would have limited her quality of life.

At age 55, she took a wrong step in the garage, and she suffered a herniated disc. The pain was breathtaking, and she was bedridden for days until she underwent a laminectomy, which is a surgical procedure to make room for the herniated disc so there is no longer compression on the nerve. The purpose of the surgery was to ease the pain of herniation, and they considered the surgery successful since her immediate pain was reduced and she was able to start working again, but her enduring pain remained.

Years later, after she entered retirement, she found herself unable to do the things she wanted to do. While she enjoyed living in a rural area, it meant she had to do a lot of physical labor to maintain her daily life. She found herself unable to do the things around the house that were necessary. Even worse, she found herself unable to do her hobbies, the things that she enjoyed, the things that made her life worth living. She was losing the feeling in her right hand and having difficulty doing her handwork. At times, the pain, along with the numbness and tingling, was so bad that she was even struggling to hold a pen long enough to sign her name. She felt her independence quickly slipping away from her.

Today, because of regenerative medicine, my mother manages a local flower shop. She quilts, crochets, sews, and makes flower arrangements, all without pain. She chops wood for her fireplace. She builds rock sidewalks for her yard. She builds fences around her house, and since she has started raising chickens, she has built a chicken coop.

I would like to say that I am such a stellar daughter that I got into medicine to fix my mother's physical problems, but that is not the case. In fact, I had no idea then that the type of medicine that would eventually capture my heart would be the medicine that changed her life and the other patients who I have had the opportunity to serve. I can't even say that I had the foresight to know that this medicine would be such a powerful force in my life on any level. I became a doctor because I had a passion for giving people options and allowing them to live out their definition of quality of life. By the grace of God, I was directed in my steps and provided with mentors who cared, listened, taught, and expanded my vision. What I found along the way were the treatments that I wholeheartedly believe in, which I have used not only on a multitude of patients but also on my mother and myself. Regenerative medicine gives hope, healing, and quality of life. It opens up treatment options that may not have been explored otherwise, and it provides opportunities that once did not exist.

Natural Therapies Meet Modern Medicine

Conventionally, the medical system has relied on suppressing symptoms, turning them off, and ignoring them rather than addressing them, supporting the body in healing, and taking the time to rest. For most people, the act of supporting the body during the healing process is one of the most difficult aspects of healing. In our society today, we don't have to wait for anything. We have microwavable meals, food delivery, Internet ordering, and drive-through service ranging from dry cleaning to banking to food service. There is nothing wrong with convenience, but we have created a society of instant gratification, and when it comes to health, this often works against us.

Let's take a fever, for example. All of us have had a fever at some point. It is the body's way to fight an infection. While there are dangerous levels of fever, most never reach that level, but we have been conditioned to think that any fever is bad and must be shut down immediately. We have become a society that is so intent on not being sick that we wear it as a badge of honor, and we don't allow the body to do what it was designed to do, which is to protect us from microbial invaders and heal. So we take medicine to stop or suppress the fever. We reach for antibiotics at the least sniffle, even though a large majority of infections are caused by viruses that are not influenced in the least by antibiotics. When we shut it down as soon as possible with medication, we subsequently shut down the process of ridding the body of the dangerous microbe, the attacker that is making us sick, whether that's bacteria, fungus, or virus. There are downstream effects to this, which are out of the scope of this book, but important nonetheless. When we think of the reason a fever exists—to kill the infection—we can see that a knee-jerk reaction to shut down the fever short-circuits our ability to heal properly.

When it comes to injuries, we do the same thing. We believe that life will stop short if we miss even one day of work or one event with our friends or family. So instead of sitting down to rest and eating properly to support healing, we run to the local pharmacy, pick up the most popular pain reliever to reduce inflammation immediately and mask pain, and continue with our day as if nothing happened. For avid sports enthusiasts and athletes, injuries are a way of life. Suppression is expected, advised, and often financially advocated. It's only when the pain becomes excruciating, when the pain medication no longer works, or when we have been in pain for so long that we can no longer ignore it that we start looking for other options. But ignoring a small injury today, suppressing it, and shutting down the healing process can lead to longer-term chronic injuries with fewer options for healing. If we had a better idea of the variety of options available to us, we might, just maybe, seek out effective and efficient treatment sooner.

Pain is the body's way to indicate that something is wrong, much like the smoke detector in your house. If you wake up at night to the screeching sound of a smoke detector, you have two options: You can take the batteries out of the smoke detector and go back to sleep, or you can call the fire department and put out the fire. The choice is yours. Do you want to turn off the pain, or do you want to address it at the root cause and deal with it once and for all?

Natural therapies meet modern medicine is a concept of combining the understanding of how the body heals naturally with medical techniques that facilitate and stimulate natural healing. Captured within this concept is a guiding methodology of identifying the underlying cause of disease and individualizing the least invasive treatment to restore health. Relying on rigorous medical training and evidence-based studies, and applying that knowledge in a way that supports the innate healing capacity that exists in the human body is the best representation of how natural therapies meet modern medicine. When medical intervention and technology are coupled with the understanding of how the body heals, the power of the medicine takes on a completely different set of healing possibilities of restoring health to the individual. The beauty of the concept lies in the application of the knowledge; it is medicine as an art and science at the same time.

PART I

Non-Surgical Options for Treating Pain

CHAPTER 1

Real Life, Real Pain, Real Results

A 59-year-old professional cowboy whose passion was rodeo was unable to get on a horse, let alone ride and rope competitively. He came into my office barely able to walk. He was having trouble sitting down in a chair and getting up from the chair. He paced around the office, obviously in pain. You could read it in his body language, in his expressions, in his eyes. He hadn't been sleeping well for several months. The pain was so bad it would either keep him awake or wake him up. He had previously undergone back surgery and a few other procedures with temporary results. Now he was pushing through his workday with the help of narcotic pain medication. His son-in-law had made a last-minute appointment for him that day because the pain was so excruciating that he didn't think he could take it much longer. He felt desperate for relief. He said to me when he entered my office, "Doc, I'm willing to try anything." As he described his pain and talked about how he could barely get through the day, let alone do the things that were burning in his heart, I was deeply moved. We discussed some treatment options, and we settled on using PRP, platelet-rich plasma, as the primary treatment. He knew there were no guarantees, but I could see the hopefulness shine in his eyes. He said, "Doc, even if I never get to ride again, if I can just get out of the pain enough to sleep, I'll be happy." Three treatments later, he came into my office and showed me a video of him roping competitively in a rodeo again. Not only was he sleeping well, but he also no longer needed pain medication, and he was back on his horse doing what he loved.

It wasn't too long ago that I was sitting in the stands, surrounded by a bevy of passionate mixed martial arts fans. The title fight, the main event, was quickly approaching. The culmination of excitement was permeating the air. The time had arrived. The fighters were called to the ring. The walk-on song, the music chosen by the fighters to be played as they enter the cage, was blaring in the arena. The announcer, in his flavorful flare, announced the two opponents, and the crowd went wild as the hometown favorite was introduced. Both athletes were inspected. Their personal ritual was completed, and both fighters were now ready to enter the cage and begin their bout. They shook hands, and the competition began. The physicality of the sport was entertaining, stomach turning, and exciting, all at the same time. It was three short rounds with three minutes of intense competition. Before the first round was complete, the winner was announced. Just four weeks prior, the champion of this fight, the winner of the main event, had been treated at my office. He had described the pain he had been experiencing in his hand and the hesitation he had felt in throwing a punch due to the pain on impact and the instability of his knee. He had felt that his knee could go in and out of place at any time. The night of the fight, there was no sign of weakness in either his wrist or knee. I couldn't help but smile as he was announced the champion of the title fight, and there was a bit of a feeling that his win was my win as well. Regenerative injection techniques have given this athlete an option to recover faster, repair injuries more effectively, and continue to compete in the sport and career of his choosing.

These stories represent the healing power encompassed in the body. When stimulating this power with the use of regenerative medicine, the results are astounding. This is why I got into medicine.

The stories pour in each and every day. Stories about how injuries and pain are affecting the lives of real people, every day. You don't need to be a professional athlete to experience pain and become intimately familiar with the limitations that are created by injuries. In fact, it's estimated that the impact of lost productivity due to pain was between $297.4 billion and $335.5 billion in 2010.[1] This represents a 386% to 448% increase in lost productivity over the previous seven years.[2] In 2005, *ABC News*, *USA Today*, and Stanford Medical Center conducted a joint survey showing that 40% of Americans experience ongoing pain that interferes with their ability to work, mood, day-to-day activity, sleep, enjoyment of life, and relationships with others.[3] In other words, the odds that you or someone close to you suffers daily from ongoing pain are quite high. Think about the people in your life. Think about yourself. Chances are, you or someone you know is currently experiencing pain. Knee pain, back pain, neck pain, and headaches are some of the most common types of pain conditions I see, but there are other types of pain that you might not think too much about and accept as the norm. Think about the ankle that aches when you try to run or swells up every time you exercise. Think about the elbow pain that nags you and affects your golf or tennis game. Think about the numbness in your fingers, the pain in your jaw, the shoulder that keeps you awake at night. All these are conditions that I have seen in my office that are affecting people's lives to one degree or another.

Let's look at the structures that may have been damaged through injury or disease.

---

1 *The Cost of Pain to Business and Society Due to Ineffective Pain Care.* (n.d.). Retrieved November 25, 2015, from http://www.painmed.org/patientcenter/cost-of-pain-to-businesses/

2 *The Cost of Pain to Business and Society Due to Ineffective Pain Care.* (n.d.). Retrieved November 25, 2015, from http://www.painmed.org/patientcenter/cost-of-pain-to-businesses/

3 ABC News, USA Today, & Stanford Medical Center. (2005, May 9). *Broad Experience with Pain Sparks a Search for Relief* [PDF file]. Retrieved December 11, 2015, from http://abcnews.go.com/images/Politics/979a1TheFightAgainstPain.pdf

Potentially Damaged Structures

Connective tissue. For the purposes of our discussion, it's important to understand the term *connective tissue*, the role it plays, and how it is affected by injury. In general, when we discuss injury, we use the term *connective tissue* to describe a set of cells or tissues that are injured. Connective tissue is formed during fetal development of the mesoderm or middle layer. Without getting too technical, mesodermal tissue forms from the multipotent cells (cells that can develop into more than one cell type) of the embryo called the mesenchyme. This distinction becomes important when we delve deeper into regenerative treatment. Mesenchymal cells give rise to all connective tissue and their cells, including bone, muscle, cartilage, tendons, ligaments, joint capsules, blood, and lymphoid cells. Connective tissue includes ligaments, tendons, muscles, and blood vessels. It creates a continuum with skin, muscle, and nerve tissue. The function of connective tissue includes giving structural support. It's what holds the body together and gives it form and function. Think bones, cartilage, ligaments, and tendons. Ligaments connect bone to bone and tendons connect muscle to bone. Without connective tissue, we wouldn't be able to stand, sit, run, dance, or do any of the many other activities we take for granted. We tend to not think too much about our connective tissue until we have pain. Then it's all we can think about.

Muscle. There are three different types of muscle cells in the body; however, our discussion will be limited to skeletal muscle. Skeletal muscle accounts for most of the voluntary muscle movement in the body. Each muscle has an origin where it starts and an insertion where it ends. Muscle movement occurs with contraction, which is when the muscle cells move the insertion closer to the origin and the muscle length is shortened, and relaxation, which is when the muscle fibers are relaxed and returned to their original length. The process of moving between contraction and relaxation of muscle fibers is what creates movement.

The voluntary movement of the muscle is easily recognized, even if we don't consciously think about the intricacies that go into muscle movement, such as action potential and voltage-gated calcium release channels. Let's take the example of flexing the bicep muscle. The flexing motion of the bicep is about a lot more than just impressing your friends or winning an arm-wrestling competition. The bicep muscle is involved in simple acts such as raising a glass of water to take a drink, picking up your kids and tossing them overhead, and carrying in bags of groceries from the car. These muscle functions are quite well known and easily understood.

What you might not realize, however, is that a fundamental part of what a muscle does is a major cause of the pain resulting from an injury. Muscles have a protective role in the body. They don't just protect the organs; they span every joint in the body. From tiny muscles in the spine to larger muscles spanning the hip, muscles do a job that most of us don't think of, let alone appreciate. Muscles provide additional support for joints and work in collaboration with ligaments and tendons to provide stability. When a joint is injured, the joint becomes unstable. To provide protection and joint stability, muscles surrounding the injured joint begin to contract, providing joint support and increased stability. With long-term and acute injury, the muscles are continuously contracted to create joint stability, which may also contribute to pain. Along with this contraction can come pinched nerves and trigger points.

Trigger points (TrPs) are a well-known source of pain. According to Davies and Davies, "Pain clinic doctors skilled at detecting and treating trigger points have found that they're the primary cause of pain roughly 75 percent of the time and they play at least a part in virtually every pain problem."[4] TrPs are very sensitive areas in

---

4 Davies, A. & Davies, C. (2013). *The Trigger Point Therapy Workbook: Your Self-Treatment Guide to Pain Relief* (3rd ed., pp. 2). Oakland, CA: Raincoast Books.

the muscle, typically the muscle belly, which, when stimulated or pressed on, will cause radiating pain. They can be responsible for pain radiating to various parts of the body such as arms, legs, and muscles in the neck contributing to headaches. A TrP is not a muscle spasm; it's a contracture in the band of the muscle. However, the same muscle contracture causing TrP pain can cause muscle spasm, and this spasm is commonly responsible for nerve impingement and pain. This explains why an injury to the low back may be felt as far down as the ankle. This is why it is important to evaluate all connecting structures when determining the best treatment for pain. TrPs have common pain patterns. As part of the treatment of a pain pattern, it's important to assess and determine how much muscle involvement is related to the pain. While pain can come from a muscle tear, which happens frequently and in varying severity, one of the most overlooked sources of pain comes from the body's natural mechanism of protection: its ongoing muscle contraction. Once stability is restored to the joint, the muscle can return to a relaxed state, thus eliminating the pain and restoring mobility.

Ligaments. A ligament is a tough connective tissue band that holds together two bones or cartilages such as in a joint. Many of us have injured ankle ligaments while playing sports, stepping off a curb, or tripping over pets or toys. Most of us are familiar with a few ligaments in the body. Ligaments are commonly associated with ankles and knees. What you might not realize is that ligaments are found throughout the body. Almost every bone in the body has ligaments attached to it. Let's take the spine, for example. The spine is comprised of 33 vertebrae, divided over different segments: cervical, thoracic, lumbar, sacral, and coccygeal. The joints between the vertebrae are supported by many ligaments that help to keep the spinal cord safe. The ligaments of the spine prevent us from turning too far right or left or extending our spine too far by limiting our ability to bend from side to side and front to back. Ligaments, in general, provide stability and keep the joint from moving too far in one direction or the other.

While ligaments are tough, they are also somewhat stretchy and can take a fair amount of force, but they too have limits. Too much force in any one direction can cause a tear or what is more technically called a rupture. Just like any other ligament, the ligaments of the spine can become injured. The extent of the rupture will be a determining factor in treatment and should be considered on a case-by-case basis. Not all ruptures require surgery, but in most cases, a complete rupture or tear of a ligament will require a surgical consult. When addressing any musculoskeletal pain, for example, during evaluation and treatment of a spinal complaint, it's important to treat ligaments as part of the treatment plan, just as when treating an ankle injury.

Tendons. Tendons are made up of connective tissue and serve the purpose of connecting muscles to bones. They are made up of a different type of connective tissue than muscle. Tendons are less vascular than muscles, which means they have fewer blood vessels supplying them with nutrients and removing waste. It also means that tendons are slower to heal than muscles; therefore, specific treatment is required to stimulate circulation to the injured area.

Tendon injuries are frequent and can be related to overuse or injury, which can range from mild overuse to full rupture. Overuse injuries are known as tendinitis or tendinosis. The major difference between tendonitis and tendinosis is that tendonitis is considered an acute injury involving inflammation, whereas tendinosis is a chronic injury involving an array of injuries from micro-tears to complete rupture. Tendonitis pain comes and goes, whereas tendinosis pain is constant and ongoing.

Cartilage. Cartilage is flexible and resistant connective tissue. There are three different types of cartilage: hyaline cartilage, elastic cartilage, and fibrocartilage, and each type serves a different purpose. We commonly think of cartilage in the knee joint, but it exists in almost every joint in the body. Bones don't fit directly together; there is an articular surface, which is usually made up of fibrocartilage acting as a shock absorber. Cartilage is smooth and slippery, like glass, and provides a gliding surface for friction-free movement of the joints.

Cartilage can be damaged through repetitive, high-impact activities such as running and jumping. Breakdown of cartilage, regardless of the joint, is known as osteoarthritis. As cartilage breaks down, the joint becomes less stable. It becomes painful and often inflamed or swollen. Wear and tear on joints is rarely symmetrical, and portions of the joint can be more widely affected. Portions of cartilage can "chip off" and become lodged in the joint, which will then cause a locking effect. For people experiencing a breakdown of cartilage, the pain can start off as intermittent and become constant over time. Regenerating even a small amount of cartilage will recreate the gliding surface, which reduces or eliminates pain and restores mobility.

The Importance of Addressing All Structures Involved

The body is wonderfully made. Muscles, cartilage, tendons, and ligaments work together to provide both mobility and stability. Together they facilitate all the movements we do—both those we think about and those we do without thinking.

This facilitation and cooperation in movements also lead to complex involvement upon injury. Because of this complexity, treating only one part of a cooperative effort results in partial treatment and reduced effectiveness of the treatment. If you, for example, have a knee injury, and you simply get an injection into the knee joint, you may experience some benefit from that. But if you don't also treat the structures surrounding the joint, supporting the joint, cooperating in movement of the joint, the muscles, ligaments, and tendons, then effectiveness of the treatment is significantly decreased.

Regenerative injection techniques are individualized, not a one-size-fits-all. For the best results, it is imperative to treat all the involved structures—all the muscles, the tendons, and the ligaments. Doing that with injection therapy requires a thorough understanding of all the structures involved, not just the obvious ones.

As a practitioner, I'm concerned with the what, when, and how of the pain you are experiencing. It's not enough to know that there is a pain in the knee or whatever the location of pain that you feel is. I need to understand the cause of pain. I ask questions such as:

- Is the pain caused by an injury?
- Is it caused by a disease?
- How long has it been hurting?
- What hurts it most?
- What relieves it?
- Are there contributing factors?
- What treatments have you tried?
- Did they work?
- Have you had imaging, such as an X-ray or MRI?
- What does your physical exam tell me?
- If there was an injury, what were you doing?
- How did you move?
- In what position was your body?

Much like a detective, I gather information and piece it all together to best determine what is going on. This information is then used to assess the type of pain, determine which structures are damaged, and decide the appropriate treatment or treatments to provide the best results. If an injection therapy is the best treatment, it's not enough just to inject into the joint or the general area of pain and call it good. Every treatment requires a thorough understanding of the pain, the affected structures, the mechanism of the injury, and the biomechanics involved during the injury.

If someone comes into my office with the complaint of knee pain, several questions run through my mind. Through history, physical exam, and imaging, I work to determine if this is a joint injury or a disease process. Are ligaments involved? Is there a breakdown of cartilage? Are trigger points of the muscle involved? What type of pain is experienced? Is it a neuropathic pain (pain caused by nerve damage), or is it a nociceptive pain (pain caused by tissue damage)? It's an important distinction because it will likely change the course of treatment and treatment goals. What treatments have been tried before and is it possible that these treatments created an injury? By getting the answers to these questions, I obtain complete and accurate information, which leads to accurate and successful treatment. By recognizing which structures are damaged and which of the supporting structures may be contributing to the pain, the effectiveness of the treatment increases significantly. Once treatment begins, the body's innate healing powers are tapped into, and the natural functioning of the immune system forges ahead to regenerate and heal the damaged structures.

I have seen patients who previously have had injection therapies of one variety or another to treat injuries but have experienced little to no benefit at all. Upon questioning, what I find in those cases is that just one area in the entire structure has been treated, while the corresponding structures have been ignored. Upon examination of the knee, for example, while injections were administered inside the joint, I often discover that both medial and lateral collateral ligaments are affected yet were not treated. Even more so, I find trigger points in the supporting muscles from the body's attempt to stabilize the joint for such a long period, and they are contributing significantly to the pain pattern that these patients feel. When all the information is taken into consideration, and the treatment is comprehensive, we get a significantly more effective treatment.

CHAPTER 2

What Is Regenerative Medicine?

When we talk about *regenerative medicine*, the discussion can get a bit heavy in places. Some people love a heavy, science-filled discussion; others will want to skip ahead as we dive into the intricacies of regenerative medicine.

According to Merriam-Webster, the word *regenerate* means to be formed or created again.[5] Every day, the body is in a constant state of regeneration. From the skin to the liver to the muscles to the heart, the body repairs, regenerates, and heals.

Regenerative medicine, according to the National Institute of Health (NIH), "is the process of creating living, functional tissues to repair or replace tissue or organ function loss due to age, disease, damage, or congenital defect."[6] Regenerative medicine is an application of knowledge utilizing specific injection techniques to regenerate, or regrow, damaged tissue. It is effective because it stimulates the body's ability to heal.

Regenerative injection techniques (RIT) are minimally invasive, low-risk treatments available to address a variety of orthopedic

---

5 Regenerate [Def. 1]. (n.d.). *Merriam Webster Online*. Retrieved December 11, 2015, from http://www.merriam-webster.com/dictionary/regenerate

6 U.S. Department of Health & Human Services (n.d.). *NIH Fact Sheets - Regenerative Medicine*. Retrieved November 25, 2015, from http://report.nih.gov/nihfactsheets/viewfactsheet.aspx?csid=62

conditions. I find myself frequently disappointed, though no longer surprised, that patients aren't given a chance to explore regenerative treatments to address their concerns on a more widespread basis. You may already be asking yourself, "Why haven't I heard of this before?" That, my friends, is the million-dollar question.

While *regenerative medicine* as a term may not be widely known outside of specific medical circles, the technology that modern-day regenerative medicine is based on has been in place for around 100 years. The U.S. Department of Health & Human Services informs us that the first forms of regenerative medicine, which occurred as early as the early 20th century, resulted in successful transplantation of bone, soft tissues, and corneas. In 1954, the first successful kidney transplant was done, followed by successful transplants of the pancreas/kidney, liver, and heart in the 1960s. The technology was expanded in the 1980s, resulting in successful heart-lung, single-lung, double-lung, and living-donor liver transplants. Today, regenerative medicine techniques are used not only in organ transplants but also in skin replacement, wound healing, and inducing bone and connective tissue growth.[7] In orthopedic use, which is the primary scope of our discussion, we have seen evidence of tissue regrowth in a variety of tissues, including ligaments, tendons, cartilage, muscles, vessels, and bone.

Phases of Healing

Injury to connective tissue can happen in several ways: trauma, accident, disease, or surgery. In any case, the body attempts to heal using the innate mechanism of healing damaged tissue. Regardless of the source of injury, including stimulation of injury through

---

7 U.S. Department of Health & Human Services (n.d.). *NIH Fact Sheets - Regenerative Medicine.* Retrieved November 25, 2015, from http://report.nih.gov/nihfactsheets/viewfactsheet.aspx?csid=62

regenerative injection, the same healing pathway is stimulated, and healing occurs in the same pattern following the same phases. This is known as the inflammatory pathway. The first phase of this pathway is the inflammatory phase, followed by the proliferative phase, and wrapped up by the remodeling phase.

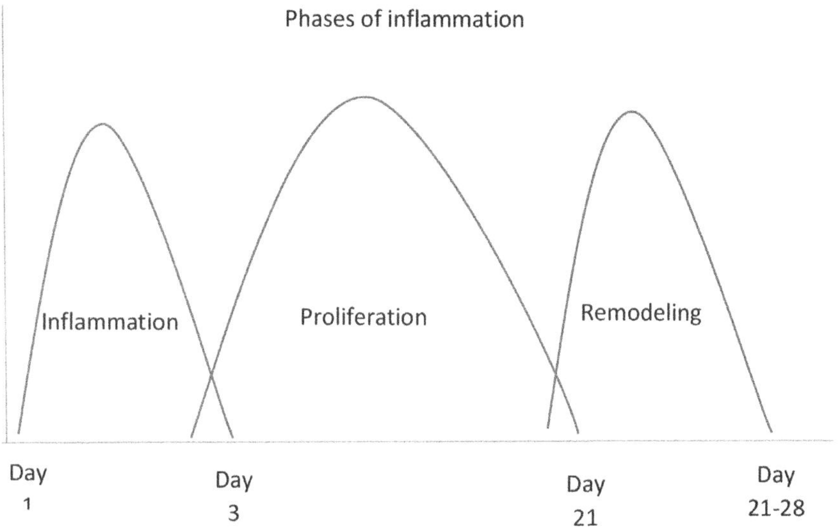

Let's look at injuries in general to understand what happens. When you injure yourself, regardless of whether it's a cut or a sprained ankle, the body follows the same basic mechanism of healing.

Inflammatory phase. During the inflammatory phase, which is the body's natural response to injury, platelets are the first responders in the immune system. That means they are the first on the scene of the injury. Initially, the vessels will contract, and platelets will form clots to stop any bleeding, otherwise known as hemostasis. The vessels in the injured area will then dilate, and that allows other cells to enter the injured area. The cells that come secondarily to the site include white blood cells, growth factors, enzymes, and nutrients that are instrumental in controlling infection, removing waste, and repairing the injury. This is the part of the process where you will likely experience swelling and pain.

Inflammation can last up to 10 days, but it typically peaks at around 24 to 48 hours after the injury or treatment. During this time, there is cell signaling called autocrine (signaling from the cell to itself) and paracrine (signaling from one cell to another) tissue factor signaling to ensure the following steps in the inflammation phase occur. This signaling ensures fibrin matrix formation (fibrin is a protein that is involved in clotting, and a fibrin matrix acts both as a sealant and scaffolding during tissue repair[8]), angiogenesis (the formation of new blood vessels from existing vessels, an intricate part of tissue healing), and production of growth factors (VEGF, PDGF, bFGF, TGFα/β, etc.) as well as adhesion molecules, all of which significantly contribute to the wound-healing process.[9]

Proliferative phase. The proliferative phase overlaps the inflammation phase and begins about three to five days after the injury or treatment. Proliferation means growth. During this phase, new granulation tissue begins to form. This granulation tissue is made up of collagen and extracellular matrix (a non-cellular component that provides scaffolding for cellular repair and initiates chemical signaling required for tissue repair and homeostasis[10]). These are the building blocks of connective tissue.

The proliferative phase continues for 21 to 28 days. During this time, new tissue is continuously forming, injured ligaments and

---

8 van Hinsbergh V.W., Collen, A., & Koolwijk, P. (2001). Role of fibrin matrix in angiogenesis. *Annals of the New York Academy of Sciences*, 936, 426–37. Retrieved from https://www.ncbi.nlm.nih.gov/pubmed/11460496

9 Chu, A.J. (2011). Tissue Factor, Blood Coagulation, and Beyond: An Overview. *International Journal of Inflammation*. Volume 2011 (2011). doi:10.4061/2011/367284

10 Frantz, C., Stewart, K. M., & Weaver, V. M. (2010). The extracellular matrix at a glance. *Journal of Cell Science*, 123(24), 4195–4200. doi:10.1242/jcs.023820

tendons are strengthening, and new vessels are forming to facilitate the transport of nutrients and the removal of waste from the injured area. Osteocytes (bone cells) and chondrocytes (cartilage cells) are also formed during this time.

During this proliferative phase, it's common to experience a waxing and waning of pain, swelling, and variable tissue strength due to the non-linear fashion that wound healing exhibits. The progression of this process is extremely individualized and can vary significantly from person to person.

Remodeling phase. The final stage of wound healing is called remodeling or maturation, depending on which source you use, and involves strengthening of collagen. Collagen is the insoluble fibrous protein of the extracellular matrix, which creates the stretchiness in connective tissue. There are at least 16 different types of collagen, but 89% to 90% of the collagen in the body is composed of collagen type 1, type 2, or type 3.

By utilizing specific injection techniques, the body is stimulated to heal injuries and restore joints, ligaments, tendons, and muscles to return the structures to their previous form and function.

The three regenerative injection techniques I would like to discuss in relation to orthopedic regenerative medicine are prolotherapy, platelet-rich plasma (also known as PRP), and stem cell therapy. It is important to understand what each type of treatment is, what it does, and any limitations or benefits it has compared to the other treatments discussed.

Prolotherapy

Prolotherapy is a regenerative injection technique recognized by the American Association of Orthopedic Medicine (AAOM) as a procedure that facilitates tissue growth and taps into the innate healing capacity of the body to restore function and mobility. Prolotherapy uses a combination of a hypertonic solution such as dextrose (a form of sugar) and an anesthetic agent such as Lidocaine or Marcaine. With precise injection techniques, the hypertonic solution and the anesthetic agent are used to target specific ligaments and tendons or injected directly into the joint to repair cartilage. The injected solution creates a mild irritation, or what we call a controlled injury. It stimulates the inflammatory process, also known as the healing cascade, and new fibrous connective tissue begins to grow in the injected area, so the injury begins to heal. The new connective tissue forms to strengthen the weakened ligaments or tendons to create a stronger, regenerated structure.

The AAOM writes about the history of prolotherapy. They cite the earliest use of a type of prolotherapy as early as 500 BC. Thankfully, science and medical technology have advanced since then. In 1926, the technique was utilized for hernias and hemorrhoids. It was furthered in orthopedic use in the 1940s and 1950s by Dr. Earl Gedney, D.O., and Dr. George Stuart Hackett, M.D.[11] Today there is strong evidence supporting prolotherapy as an effective nonsurgical treatment for a variety of musculoskeletal injuries.

Platelet-Rich Plasma

Platelet-rich plasma (PRP) is a nonsurgical regenerative treatment used to speed proliferation, or regrowth, and healing of injured or damaged structures, much like prolotherapy. The injection technique of PRP is similar to prolotherapy. However, the solution injected is quite different. Platelet-rich plasma is an autologous solution that is created using the patient's own blood. We draw a few vials of blood and spin it down a couple of times using a specific centrifugation

11 AAOM. (2013). Prolotherapy FAQs. Retrieved December 1, 2015, from http://www.aaomed.org/Injection-Therapy-FAQ

process to separate out the red and white blood cells. We pitch the red cells and keep the plasma cells, which are further processed at a high G-force to separate the platelets from the plasma. We then throw away about two-thirds of the plasma and reconstitute or resuspend the platelets in the remaining plasma, resulting in a high concentration of platelets with a little bit of plasma—platelet-rich plasma. At this point, we inject that PRP into specific locations of injury and pain. Once PRP is injected, the body goes to work immediately.

Platelets play a key role in wound healing. They are sticky, and they help to prevent blood loss and vascular injury. Think about if you were to cut yourself on the hand. They rush to the area to aggregate, or clump together, to first stop the bleeding. But they also send signals to the immune system, called chemotaxis, to call growth factors to the area so that healing can begin. Since platelets are sticky, they adhere to and aggregate to create the surface that promotes thrombin and fibrin formation. Without these growth factors, a cut would never close, nerves and muscle would not repair, and frankly most of us would never have made it out of childhood.

Platelets release active proteins and metabolites that create tissue factor signaling. The tissue factor signaling initiates inflammation, along with interleukins that bind to developing fibrin, one of the components of connective tissue and extracellular matrix. This binding creates a chemotactic gradient that recruits stem cells to the area. Platelets "turn on" the stem cells, causing them to migrate and differentiate, which promotes repair. The fibrin clot that is used by the platelets promotes rapid healing. When we inject PRP into an injured area, we are stimulating the inflammation process to happen. While systemic inflammation is not healing, local inflammation is required for healing. So we get an inflammatory response for 24 to 48 hours after injection—some dull aching, possible swelling, maybe a little heat—all signs of inflammation. After the initial inflammatory phase is complete, with some overlapping, we get the proliferation phase. During this time, tissues are regenerating, healing, and getting stronger.

Studies show that PRP is effectively used in dental implant surgery, orthopedic surgery, muscle and tendon repair, skin ulcers, eye surgery, and cardiac surgery where the use of autologous platelets will accelerate healing.[12]

Stem Cell Therapy

Adult stem cells are stem cells that are formed during the development of the fetus and remain in the body throughout the rest of the person's life.[13] There are different types of stem cells. Totipotent cells can form any type of cells in the body and extraembryonic, or placental, cells. Embryonic cells are cells that are formed within the first couple of divisions after fertilization, the only true totipotent cells. Pluripotent cells can form any type of cell in the body. Embryonic stem cells are considered pluripotent. Multipotent cells can develop into more than one type of cell but are limited. Adult stem cells and cord blood (umbilical) stem cells are both multipotent.[14] There are different types of adult stem cells that can be used for therapeutic purposes: bone marrow derived, which are stem cells stored in the bone marrow, and adipose derived, which are stem cells stored in the fat. In this context, we will be discussing adipose-derived autologous stem cell therapy utilizing mesenchymal-derived adult stem cells.

---

12 Nurden, A., Nurden, P., Sanchez, M., Andia, I., & Anitua, E. (2008). Platelets and wound healing. *Frontiers in bioscience :bioscience: a Journal and Virtual Library,* 13, 3532–48. Retrieved February 3, 2017, from https://www.ncbi.nlm.nih.gov/pubmed/18508453

13 A Closer Look at Stem Cells (2015). *Nine Things to Know About Stem Cell Treatments.* Retrieved December 1, 2015, from http://www.closerlookatstemcells.org/stem-cells-and-medicine/nine-things-to-know-about-stem-cell-treatments

14 New York State Stem Cell Science (n.d.). *What is the difference between totipotent, pluripotent, and multipotent?* Retrieved February 3, 2017, from https://stemcell.ny.gov/faqs/what-difference-between-totipotent-pluripotent-and-multipotent

Mesenchymal stem cells, also known as MSC, are multipotent, meaning they have the ability to differentiate into multiple types of cells, including bone cells (osteocytes), cartilage cells (chondrocytes), muscle cells (myocytes), and other types of connective tissue. In other words, mesenchymal stem cells become any cell that needs to be repaired—except blood cells.

According to the National Stem Cell Foundation:

> Adipose (fat) tissue is one of the richest sources of mesenchymal stem cells. There are about 500 times more mesenchymal stem cells in 1 gram of fat than there are in 1 gram of bone marrow.[15]

The stem cells are harvested by a liposuction technique to obtain the patient's own adipose stroma or fat. The cells are then minimally manipulated utilizing technology to isolate the stem cells. At this point, they are known as a stromal vascular fraction (SVF). The SVF is then injected into the patient to treat the particular condition. Studies have shown that 95% of adipose-derived mesenchymal stem cells will become new tissue. We can achieve a therapeutic benefit by infusing as few as 10 million stem cells. Obviously, the larger the harvest, the larger the therapeutic benefit will be. For example, a harvest of between 60 milliliters and 100 milliliters of adipose will theoretically yield an estimated 60 million to 100 million stem cells for reinfusion.

Both stem cell therapy and PRP therapy have been in use since the 1990s, and they are both used to treat a variety of conditions, specifically orthopedic injuries. Each of these treatments works in a common healing pathway or a healing cascade, given the cascade of events that occurred to create healing and regeneration of tissue.

Over the next few chapters, we will look further into various conditions and which treatment methods may be suited for these.

---

15 NSCF (2015). *Mesenchymal Stem Cells.* Retrieved December 1, 2015, from http://www.nationalstemcellfoundation.org/mesenchymal-stem-cells/

CHAPTER 3

Choosing the Right Tool

Western medicine and the type of medicine we practice conventionally in the United States often discount the body's amazing healing power. Many people have been conditioned to think that if a treatment doesn't include prescription drugs or surgery, the body can't take care of itself. That is not to say that prescription drugs and surgery aren't useful because they are when used in the proper context. The technological advances we have had in both pharmaceuticals and surgery over the past hundred years have been astounding.

It is, however, important to remember that pharmaceuticals and surgery are tools. Choosing the right tool for the condition at hand is paramount for the treatment to be effective. Luckily, with the way that I have been trained in medicine, I have a lot of tools at my disposal and can select the appropriate one for the condition of the patient sitting in front of me.

Sometimes surgery is the best option. I am more than happy to refer a patient to someone else when that is appropriate. Not one single person in medicine is going to have all the answers all the time. It's important to explore your options for treating and healing the injury or disease process that is affecting your body.

While regenerative injection techniques have been well studied and used successfully for several years, there are some who are not yet acquainted with the procedures. The most common objections I hear to these techniques include "My family doctor says they don't work" and "My doctor says they are not well studied." Unfortunately, a doctor who makes this type of comment is not up to date on the literature and studies that have proven that regenerative medicine works. I wouldn't expect a primary care doctor to be caught up on the literature of regenerative medicine or orthopedic medicine because that is not what he or she specializes in. But the truth is that prolotherapy, PRP, and stem cell treatment are both effective and well studied.

Efficiency can vary between techniques because the technology and the science behind them differ. We can think about it in levels. Prolotherapy would be the first level. Then a more efficient treatment for injuries would be PRP, so that would be the second level. Then the third level would be stem cells, which would be an even more efficient, and in many cases, more effective treatment. Depending on the injury and other individualizing factors, the doctor performing the treatment should be able to help you determine the treatment that will be most effective and efficient for you. It's not that one treatment is not going to get you to the end goal, which would be return of function, return of form, and reduction of pain. But it may take longer to get there with prolotherapy because it's not as efficient a procedure as PRP. While prolotherapy is a viable, effective treatment, because technology has improved, we now have treatments that are more efficient.

As a practitioner, of the three regenerative techniques discussed, I generally use PRP more often than either prolotherapy or stem cell therapy. In many cases, the cost of stem cell therapy is prohibitive for patients, and in some cases, stem cell therapy is overkill for the injury at hand. I work with my patients to determine the most efficient, effective treatment given all the constraints. When it comes down to it, PRP is both effective and efficient while being within the budget of the majority of patients.

During my evaluation of a patient, I look at the whole picture to gain information needed to make a good decision. That is a cornerstone of my practice. Physical exams are an essential part of the evaluation. We can gain a lot of information just by doing a physical exam. But I have patients come to my office stating that many, if not all, of the doctors they have been to in search of treatment for their pain did little to no physical exam at all. Touching the patient to gather information seems to be a dying art.

Years ago, the physical exam was commonly the only diagnostic tool the doctor would use. Imaging, such as X-rays, MRIs, and CT scans, weren't widely available and were very cost prohibitive for many people. Fortunately for us, diagnostic imaging is readily available now, and with a bit of legwork, it can be reasonably priced for those who need to pay out-of-pocket. The downside, however, is that with increasing availability of diagnostic imaging, it seems many doctors solely rely on the image instead of pairing the imaging with the physical exam to obtain a complete picture, thereby losing the benefit of the hands-on physical exam.

I utilize physical exams, diagnostic imaging, and medical history. I take that information and piece it together to complete the puzzle of the patient's health. In some cases, I also order blood tests to fill in gaps or answer questions that I am unable to answer without them. Once I have put together all the pieces, I can accurately assess the proper treatment for the individual patient.

Factors That Influence Healing

The factors that influence healing from regenerative treatments are similar to the factors that influence innate healing (healing that occurs naturally without surgical or regenerative intervention) at the time of the injury.

Factors that can influence the effectiveness of regenerative treatments include the following:

- Age
- Overall health
- Preexisting medical conditions
- Autoimmune diseases
- Scarring issues such as hypertrophic scars or keloid scars
- Hormone balance
- Nutrition
- The severity of the injury
- The length of time since injury—how long ago the injury or pain occurred
- Smoking status—smokers tend to heal more slowly than non-smokers. A lot of oxidation occurs in the body as a result of smoking, and it can impede the healing process.

All the above factors will influence the effectiveness of any of the regenerative medicine treatments. We see a similar reduction in healing time for those who have diabetes because the disease impedes overall wound healing and circulation. How much influence these factors will have is a discussion to have with the doctor performing the treatment. Some of these will have little influence while others will have more significant influence. Again, each person seeking treatment is an individual and has to be assessed as an individual. There is not one cut-and-dried set of what works and what doesn't work. The results of each type of treatment are likely to vary based on the individual, and the risks and benefits associated with each type of treatment should be discussed with the doctor performing the treatment before the treatment takes place.

There are a few people who are not good candidates for regenerative medicine. Patients who have diseases that are treated with immunosuppressive drugs, such as prednisone or cortisone, are not good candidates for regenerative medicine while they are on the medication. This is due to the nature of the treatment. Since regenerative injection techniques rely on an immune system response, when the immune system has been suppressed by drugs, it will not respond, therefore creating an ineffective treatment. Any drug that directly influences the inflammatory pathway that regenerative medicine relies on to create new tissue will also suppress the effectiveness of the regenerative treatment. Patients treated with prednisone and other steroids must allow the medication to be metabolized out of the body and follow a proper wean-down process. It can take anywhere from a few to several weeks as the medications cannot be stopped abruptly. A physician can help them safely wean off the medication. After that has taken place, there is usually no problem beginning any of the regenerative treatments. Patients who have received a recent cortisone shot to ease pain might not be able to proceed with the treatment until that medication is out of the system. However, there are occasions where a local treatment of a steroid is used in one part of the body but not taken orally. Depending on the area of treatment, it might be possible to proceed with the treatment in a different area of the body. A physician can make the appropriate recommendation regarding treatments following steroid injection.

It is the same for patients who are treated with nonsteroidal anti-inflammatory drugs (NSAID). NSAIDs include over-the-counter medicine (OTC) such as Aspirin, Motrin (ibuprofen), Aleve, and Excedrin. It can also be prescription medication such as naproxen, meloxicam, diclofenac, fenoprofen, and many others. While the medication is in their system, the inflammatory pathway needed to create proliferation of connective tissue, as discussed in Chapter 2, is blocked. For patients who are undergoing these treatments, we have to wait until the medication is no longer in the body. For NSAIDs, the half-life (the time required for a substance or drug to lose half of its effectiveness in the body) is quite short. By 24 to 48 hours, the NSAIDs are completely out of the system, so for such medication, I suggest waiting 24 hours.

There are a few other conditions that are not well suited for regenerative medicine. One of those is broken bones. Broken bones may need to be set properly in order to heal correctly. Patients need to go to the emergency room or an orthopedic doctor for that. I'm not the right type of doctor to come to for setting a broken bone. While there are treatments I use in-office to speed the healing of a broken bone, regenerative medicine isn't typically the treatment I determine to be the best fit.

The Need for Patience After Treatment

Regenerative medicine does not provide overnight healing. It is very important to manage expectations. Patients sometimes think that the pain will immediately resolve and not return after getting a regenerative treatment. However, that is not the way it works because that is not the way the body works. When we use pharmaceutical drugs as an option to treat pain, we will usually get the pain under control immediately and can maintain that pain control. When we go in and heal damaged areas with regenerative medicine, we rely on the body to heal, and the body does not heal overnight. If you cut your finger, it takes a few days for that cut to heal. That is the type of healing that is important to keep in mind. Depending on the injury, and especially as a part of a disease process, healing won't happen immediately. The idea is to facilitate the body's natural healing capacity and allow it to do what it naturally does, which is to restore function, increase mobility, and heal the injured area.

It's very common to experience pain throughout the course of treatment. That doesn't mean that healing is not occurring, because it is. The pain doesn't necessarily go away until the healing is complete. I see this over and over. Many people will use pain as the sole measure of healing, and it can be frustrating for patients to feel like they are not getting better. But healing is happening. Their range of motion is improving. Their strength is restored. If the pain doesn't decrease immediately after treatment, they mistakenly think that it isn't working, and they discontinue treatment.

Another mistake some make is to resume training too quickly. This is especially common amongst athletes. Athletes are some of the most impatient patients I see. I say that with all the love in my heart. For many athletes, taking time away from their sport is worse than the pain of their injury. Recently, a 35-year-old male came to my office with a labral tear in the shoulder from an injury he sustained in mixed martial arts training. He is a former competitor in the sport. Now he just fights for pleasure and fitness, but he trains and spars just as if he were training for competition. After the first treatment, his shoulder was feeling better, so he decided to work out. I received a call from him a couple of weeks after the treatment, and he asked, "Doc, could I have torn the new tissue in my shoulder by working out too soon?" The answer is yes. You have to love these guys and their dedication to the sport and their discipline. It's amazing. But their ability to abstain from aggressive training long enough to heal an injury proves to be a formidable opponent. When activity or training is resumed too quickly, the original injury can escalate quickly in severity. It doesn't matter whether you are a competitive athlete, a weekend athlete, or a person going about your regular day and regular fitness routine. If you start exercising too aggressively or too quickly with an injury that has just been treated, there is a possibility of reinjuring yourself and subsequently making the original injury worse than it was when we started.

With respect to regenerative medicine, the new tissue begins to grow within three to five days following the treatment, and it will continue to grow for three to four weeks. The new tissue doesn't have the strength of fully formed tissue, and it's subject to injury with a lower amount of force than what mature tissue would be able to sustain. Keeping this in mind, exercising with good judgment and a bit of patience go a long way to preventing re-injury and ensuring the best outcome and healing of the original injury.

Sometimes people will comment, "I have had injection therapies, and they didn't work for me. I spent a lot of money and didn't get any benefit." We never reach 100% return after an injury, even with successful treatment or surgery. There was an injury, and we can repair it, but we can't erase it. Assuming treatment is completed, and there are no extenuating circumstances, success rates in my office are high. The majority of people will return to close to 95% function, and they will be pain-free and able to walk, exercise, and work without pain.

Injury and disease are no respecter of persons. They happen to the young and the old, to the active and the inactive, to the athlete and the spectator. All of us will, at some point in life, experience the pain of injury or disease. While there are contributing factors to healing and recovery, I see results in a wide variety of patients, male and female, young and old. The youngest patient I have treated was a 9-year-old athlete. The oldest was a 96-year-old grandmother who loved to attend martini and pie-baking parties with her granddaughter. Her goal was to be able to stand long enough to bake a pie and walk around the block every once in a while. Every patient—from symptoms to treatment goals—is different. Since we are using the body's ability to heal, we are not limited in the number of treatments we can do. Depending on the treatment goals, we can vary the aggressiveness of the treatment, or we can stretch it out. The bottom line is that I meet you where you are and treat you until you are happy with the results.

CHAPTER 4

Musculoskeletal Pain

When we ask who can benefit from regenerative treatment, the answer is almost anybody. Regenerative medicine is not a one-size-fits-all treatment, but there are many different applications for it. A wide variety of conditions and patients can receive benefit from the regenerative techniques whether it is PRP, prolotherapy, or stem cell therapy.

When it comes to musculoskeletal pain, prolotherapy, PRP, and stem cell therapy work well. How is it that these three types of regenerative treatments can be utilized for so many people? Given the fact that everybody is different, how can we use the treatments the same way for so many different people and so many varieties of injuries? It's very simple. Regenerative therapy taps into the healing system that is already in place—the immune system. Because we are tapping into the innate healing capacity of the body, a sophisticated system by design, a system that is inherently versatile, we get to utilize the benefit of the versatility.

Now let us turn our attention to what injuries can be treated with regenerative medicine. Sometimes people are greatly surprised to learn that we have such a wide variety of uses for regenerative medicine.

Headache and Jaw Pain

Headaches can be debilitating as anyone who suffers from them can attest. One of the treatments I use for headaches is PRP. While there are multiple causes of headaches, soft tissue injury to the neck should not be overlooked. Soft tissue injury can be caused by trauma such as a motor vehicle accident, sports relates injuries, or degenerative disorders. Headaches can also be caused by a common chronic disorder known as TMJ syndrome, which creates jaw pain that radiates through the entire face and over the head. The temporomandibular joint (TMJ) is a small, fragile joint, subject to injury from trauma, grinding teeth, and degenerative processes just like any other joint. As a sports-related injury, it can be due to a blow to the jaw such as in boxing, MMA (mixed martial arts), and gymnastics. It's about getting to the root cause. The pain in TMJ syndrome is caused by ligament laxity and in some cases, degeneration of the joint.

Ligament laxity is just a fancy name for a strained ligament. When two bones fit together, it's what we call articulation. Any time a bone articulates with another bone, there is a ligament that attaches over the joint to help stabilize and hold that joint in place. When that ligament is stretched, strained, or sprained, we get ligament laxity. It's similar to taking a rubber band and stretching it over and over again. Eventually it loses elasticity and becomes lax. Ligament laxity, whether that joint is the elbow or somewhere along the spine, causes the same problem of an unstable joint, which can lead to pain, numbness, and tingling. It can also lead to progressive types of compensatory injuries, meaning another part of the body compensates for the initial injury, which causes an injury there. It's not uncommon for the compensatory injury to cause as much or more pain than the initial injury.

I have also had people come in with what they describe as face pain, where they have pain along the nerves of their face, over their cheek or forehead. I have utilized different types of regenerative medicine techniques to combat that face pain. In many cases, I manage to remove the pain completely, and that makes a huge difference in their lives.

Neck Pain

The neck is a very commonly injured area. Neck pain can be caused by a variety of things like vertebral misalignment, muscle strains, and ligament sprains, just to mention a few. We can also get herniated discs in the neck. People tend to associate herniated discs with the lower back, and though that is a common area of disc herniation, a herniation can occur anywhere along the spine. I quite frequently see herniation of the cervical spine (the neck). That will often lead to numbness and tingling from the arms all the way down to the fingers. Some might even have lost their mobility to the point where they are unable to write, do handwork or crafts, or do other activities that involve fine motor skills of their fingers. When we address the issue, those symptoms resolve. The tingling they have experienced is eliminated, and the feeling in their fingers and mobility is restored so that they can begin to use their hands again. Addressing the problem in the neck is key to solving the problem.

Recent literature has documented the connection of chronic neck pain with ligament laxity and cervical instability. Ligament laxity allows for excessive movement of the cervical spine. Depending on the area of the spine where ligament laxity occurs, a variety of symptoms can be felt. These symptoms include face pain, arm pain, vertigo, (a feeling that the world is spinning around or you are spinning around in the world), headaches, nerve irritation, numbness, and muscle spasm, which can be quite significant. By addressing ligament laxity, we can stabilize the joints in the vertebrae of the neck, and we will see results such as decreased pain, restored mobility, and returned function, not to mention improved quality of life.

Many people have whiplash injuries to the neck that they don't even know of. Whiplash can involve both muscle strain and ligament sprain. While there are times that during injury, ligament strain and disc herniation will occur concurrently, the more common injury is for years' worth of ligament strain and laxity to occur before disc herniation. Longstanding whiplash injuries can lead to a progression of chronic headaches. Fixing the whiplash injury is paramount in eliminating head and neck pain.

Motor vehicle accidents are very common. It doesn't even have to be a major accident for those involved to warrant treatment. Even injuries from a fender-bender can cause excruciating pain for years after the accident. A 35-year-old female came to my office with low back pain and neck pain that she got from an injury in a car accident. At the time I started seeing her, she had been seeing a chiropractor three times a week for six months. She told me that after those visits, she would feel better for a day or so, but the relief would not last. She was very frustrated because she had a young child at home, and she wasn't able to play with him and carry him around like she needed and wanted to due to the pain. She had been controlling the pain with prescription pain medicine, but she didn't want to continue with this treatment long term. After the first treatment of PRP, she was able to decrease her pain medication, although she still needed it for occasional relief. After three treatments on her low back, the treatment of that area was complete. She no longer had any pain in that area, and she no longer took pain medication. She did still have an occasional headache from the neck tightness and the neck pain. The pain was about 80% better than what it had been when we started the treatments, and she no longer saw the chiropractor. After two additional treatments focused on her neck, the neck pain was completely resolved, and she was released to full activity.

I'm a big supporter of chiropractic care. In my office, I use naturopathic manipulation techniques that are very similar to chiropractic care, and I have been taken care of by some amazing chiropractors my entire life. But in this case, chiropractic care just wasn't the right tool to repair the damage. Again, it's about choosing the right tool for the injury. Since this patient wasn't getting the expected benefit from chiropractic care, her chiropractor referred her to me for additional treatment.

Shoulder Pain

In my office, I commonly see an array of shoulder injuries that are very effectively treated by all three of the regenerative techniques we have talked about. It includes injuries to the rotator cuff (the muscles that hold the arm onto the shoulder girdle), acromioclavicular (AC) joint injuries, various types of tendonitis, and even labral tears. A labral tear is considered a more significant injury. The labrum is a small cartilage-like cuff that sits in the joint of the shoulder. It is similar to a meniscus in the knee. The labrum tear is much like a cartilage tear, so we rebuild it the same way we rebuild cartilage. I have used both PRP and stem cells very successfully to treat labral tears. When PRP gets in there, especially with a labral tear or a meniscal tear, it acts like glue. The sticky platelets in PRP help knit the tear back together.

Shoulder injuries, in general, are the injuries that take the longest to heal—or they feel like they take the longest to heal, with the ankle as a close second. It seems to take so long to heal because of the amount of movement of the shoulder. We use it for everything.

Elbow Pain

People can have elbow pain from the ligaments on the inside and the outside of the elbow. They may have tennis elbow, golfer's elbow, or any tendonitis in the elbow. There are also more severe injuries like Tommy John injuries, which are often but not exclusively associated with baseball players. (Fun fact: This type of injury was named after the baseball player Tommy John.) Others who typically get these injuries are MMA fighters, jiu-jitsu fighters, and boxers. These are injuries to the ulnar collateral ligament in the elbow and are typically considered surgical. However, I have seen both stem cell and PRP procedures produce some amazing results in the treatment of the more common tendonitis or tendinosis type of injuries and the less common injuries like Tommy John injuries.

Wrist and Hand Pain

Wrist and hand injuries, carpal tunnel syndrome, numbness and tingling in the hands, and deformed or swollen joints from diseases like rheumatoid arthritis are all conditions that have been successfully treated. If you have fallen and caught yourself, your hand or wrist may continue to ache. This is typically due to ligament injury and can be successfully treated with RIT.

Low Back, Sacroiliac Joint, and Sciatic Pain

Back pain is one of the most common causes of lost work and wages. The general term *low back pain* can include pain in the lumbar spine, paraspinal muscles of the lumbar spine, or sacroiliac joint. In some cases, pain in the low back can refer down the back of the leg from the gluteal region to the knee or foot. This referral pain is referred to as sciatic pain due to the impingement of the sciatic nerve. This pain can be caused by herniated discs, muscle spasm in the paraspinal muscles of the lumbar spine, joint degeneration, nerve impingement, spinal stenosis, and other soft tissue injuries.

It's important to realize that pain might not come from where it is felt; it might be a referral pain from an injury elsewhere. It's important to assess, and this is where the physical exam comes in.

Hip Pain

Sometimes the pain that is referred to as hip pain is actually low back pain. It's important to properly assess the region of pain and understand how the structures work together to create movement. When this happens, accurate assessment of pain-generating structures allows for proper treatment. When there is hip pain, the hip labrum may be involved. When the labrum is torn, it often feels like the joint is unstable, like it's going to give out with use or pressure. The pain caused by a labral tear can be quite significant. I have seen patients with labral tears who have undergone surgical procedures and nerve ablation to try to eliminate the pain. One patient had undergone a nerve ablation—they had gone in and burned the nerves of the leg—rather than fix the labrum in the hip joint itself. In that case, the patient's pain never subsided, and it ended up causing her more pain and discomfort. Unfortunately, she wouldn't undergo any regenerative medicine techniques, so I wasn't able to show her the benefit of getting the labrum fixed.

When it comes to the hip, I also see a lot of kicking injuries. These are usually, but not exclusively, sports-related. Soccer players or people who do karate or mixed martial arts—people who do a lot of kicking action—have the propensity to get tendonitis in a hip flexor, which can cause pain in the groin. Now, there are a lot of reasons for pain in the groin, but one of the things that should be assessed is tendonitis or tendinosis.

Again, whenever there is an injury to tendons or ligaments, regenerative treatments are excellent alternatives to surgery. Sometimes, even with hip pain, we see a referral pattern around to the front of the hip or into the groin area. It will come from the hip whether it's a problem in the hip joint or in the hip socket itself, like a labral tear, or a problem with the ligaments that attach to the top of the femoral head. All the major stabilizing muscles in the back of the body —gluteus medius, gluteus maximus, and gluteus minimus—connect from the top of the hipbone (iliac crest) down to the greater trochanter, which is the top of the leg, or what we usually call the hip. It's not inside but outside the joint. When the tendons connecting these muscles to the bone are affected, we get a pain that takes a variety of radiation patterns and can cause difficulty walking, bending, or even sleeping. It can be very painful to lie on that side. When sleeping aggravates any pain, regardless of the area of the body, we get into a catch 22 situation: Lack of sleep exacerbates the pain, and the pain keeps us from sleeping. It can feel like a never-ending cycle.

Knee Injuries

Many people have knee injuries. These injuries can come from overuse, stepping wrong, twisting the ankle, twisting the knee, or sports injuries. They can also come as part of a disease process. I see knee injuries like meniscal tears and tendon and ligament injuries, degenerative arthritic conditions, and generalized knee pain. There are a multitude of structures in and around the knee joint that can be injured. Knee pain can vary from specific activity induced pain, to constant pain. Patients will often cite difficulty walking, sleeping, and working as a result of a knee injury. Fortunately, knees typically respond well to RIT.

Foot and Ankle Injuries

Many of my patients come to me with foot and ankle injuries. Since I see many athletes, I often encounter a condition called Turf Toe, which is a sprain of a ligament in the foot. It is a common condition among football players, MMA fighters, tennis players, and soccer players—anybody who stops abruptly.

Then there is plantar fasciitis. Plantar fasciitis seems to go from the very active to the moderately active to the low-activity population. Plantar fasciitis is an inflammation of the tendons of the foot, a tendinopathy if you will. It can be treated the same as any other tendinopathy in the body and responds well to regenerative treatment.

One often overlooked cause of plantar fasciitis is an injury to the sacroiliac joint of the spine. Spraining these ligaments can cause an indirect or compensatory injury of the foot that is often diagnosed as plantar fasciitis.

Then there are sprains and strains in the ankle. It's quite easy to sprain the ankle. You can twist it just by doing an exercise or stepping off the curb wrong. I see a lot of ankle strains, both acute and chronic injuries. It's common for an ankle to remain swollen for years after the initial injury. It remains weak and is overly susceptible to re-injury.

I even receive patients with bunions. I have successfully treated bunions with PRP, reducing the abnormal bone growth and allowing people to wear regular shoes again.

Those are many of the types of injuries that I encounter and have been able to treat with regenerative medicine, but it is by far not an exhaustive list.

CHAPTER 5

Arthritic Conditions

Arthritic conditions are very well served by regenerative injection techniques. Osteoarthritis, rheumatoid arthritis, and psoriatic arthritis are some of the more common arthritic conditions that can be helped with these techniques. Each of these arthritic conditions has a different cause. In order to treat the condition effectively, it's important to treat the cause of the condition and help the body heal the damage. Let's talk about these conditions.

Rheumatoid Arthritis

Rheumatoid arthritis (RA) is an arthritic condition caused by an autoimmune disease. In any autoimmune disease, the immune system, in a simplistic view, gets confused and begins to attack normal tissue as if it were a pathogen or something that needs to be destroyed. In RA, joints are deformed, swollen, painful, and often damaged to the point of immobility. I have seen patients who experience deformity to such an extreme degree that they have difficulty performing what can be considered mundane activity such as buttoning buttons or opening doors with knobs. When the fingers are affected, we can lose a great deal of independence. When toes are affected, we can lose the ability to comfortably wear shoes and walk.

A 50-year-old male came into my office as a new patient. He had been diagnosed with RA a few years prior. For several years, he had managed to keep his condition under control by modifying his diet. Then, eight months prior to coming to me, he started feeling pain, and it was escalating. (The pain that comes with RA can wax and wane, so sometimes it will be fine, and other times it will flare up and be debilitating.) He was under the care of a rheumatologist and had tried several different types of medication to control the pain and reduce the flare. Some of the medication had a slight effect, but most of it had none at all. He had also tried some alternative treatments like acupuncture and herbs, but still he had not been able to break the flare. He was just miserable. If you have RA, or you are close to somebody who has RA, you know what I mean by miserable. He wasn't able to sleep. He was losing weight. He was having difficulty walking. He was very afraid that he was about to lose his job because his mobility was significantly affected by his arthritis. Unfortunately, stress can have a negative impact on RA. While this patient had a flare going on, he was afraid that he would lose his job, and he was stressed out about that. Stress, whether it's physiological stress, which is stress in the body, or psychological stress, which is stress we might feel from a family or work situation, exacerbates and keeps the flare going. So all the things that were going on were not helping his condition. I felt deeply for him.

When he came to my office, he was no longer on any medication, and he was hoping PRP treatment might help him. However, he was in the midst of a flare, and his pain was in every joint of his body from his fingers to his toes. I had to ask myself: If I were to use PRP, where would I inject it to get any benefit? Since it wasn't obvious which joint I would attack using this treatment, I had to determine that he wasn't a great candidate for PRP at this point. Once we were able to get his RA under control and manage his flare, then we could make some strategic decisions about utilizing PRP. We did discuss stem cell therapy as an option to treat the autoimmune condition to break the flare and heal the gut, the source of autoimmunity. In this case, the cost of the treatment was prohibitive. Because of this patient's situation, I suggested a different treatment to manage the symptoms and begin the healing process. Then we had the option of discussing regenerative injections at a later time. The treatment goals for him were to minimize his pain and reduce his flare immediately and then begin to heal his gut. The gut is the root of almost every autoimmune condition, which is what RA is. We broke it down to the most basic healing techniques: we addressed nutritional imbalances, supported his immune system, healed his gut, and changed much of his daily routine including the foods he ate. With this strategy, although the results were slower, over a couple of years, we have been able to rid him of the pain, prevent further progression of the disease, and give him back the quality of life that he was missing. As the flare resolves, we are better equipped to assess the damaged joints and start working on repairing those joints and any joint deformity that may have come as a result of the disease.

While we didn't utilize any of the regenerative injection techniques with this patient, I share this story with you for two purposes: to demonstrate the variety of treatments that can be effective, and to demonstrate the importance to me as a physician to find the treatment that works with the patients, where they are when they come to me. I find no satisfaction in performing ineffective treatments for the sake of money. It's about my integrity as a provider and a person. If I recommend a treatment, I do so with the whole-hearted belief that the treatment will be effective for the patient in front of me. It's how I would want to be treated if I were sitting in the patient's position.

I tend not to jump right to regenerative treatments for someone who has rheumatoid arthritis and is in an acute flare unless we are considering stem cells to get it under control. Stem cells will attack the root cause of the autoimmune disease. Therefore, this type of treatment can be used immediately. It repairs the cause of the autoimmunity, influences the inflammation, and begins to repair the joints. I have used stem cells in cases of an acute flare. They are effective and efficient as a treatment even then. In many cases of an acute flare, it's probably one of the best treatment options. It doesn't have to be used as a sole treatment, but it can be used as a part of a comprehensive treatment plan. Again, it's about selecting the proper treatment for the patient in front of me. Even with similar disease processes, there might be different answers to which is the best treatment to utilize at the particular time.

Due to a different mechanism of action, PRP is usually not used immediately to repair joints while a patient is in an acute flare. But there have been times where I have used PRP for an acute flare when it involved one or two joints because we do get the benefit of shifting inflammation as well as joint repair, which results in relief. Many people I see who are in their initial stages of treatment with RA are in a state of inflammation that is so diffuse that every joint is painful. Then the question becomes, like I said earlier, what joint do I treat to get results? If I am unable to definitively answer that, I use another treatment initially, and then I revisit PRP or prolotherapy as a long-term treatment strategy. Though PRP is not the best treatment for a person who has an acute RA flare, it is effective to correct the damage caused by RA. The individual and their particular situation have to be taken into account, and then a sound, clinical decision has to be made based on that.

Psoriatic Arthritis

Psoriatic arthritis is a chronic inflammatory arthritis that can vary in severity ranging from occasional flares of pain to joint damage. It is seen in association with psoriasis, an autoimmune disease, but may or may not accompany the more commonly known skin rash. As with all joint deformity caused by autoimmune disease, the underlying cause needs to be addressed prior to treating joint deformity, and during an acute inflammatory state, prolotherapy and PRP would not be recommended. Stem cell therapy is the better option for addressing both joint damage and autoimmune disease, even during an acute flare.

Osteoarthritis

Osteoarthritis is a condition caused by overuse. Our joints take a beating as we live our lives. I've heard osteoarthritis described as "the consequence of living an active lifestyle." Many people accept their joint damage as "just part of getting older." From one perspective, I suppose this is true; the body begins breaking down from the moment we are born, and certainly healing and recovery come more slowly as the years tick on, but it doesn't relegate us to a life of no choices, to living in pain.

The mechanism of osteoarthritis is different from rheumatoid arthritis. Whereas rheumatoid arthritis is an autoimmune disease, osteoarthritis is a degenerative disease. At the end of each bone in the body, there is a protective cartilage. That cartilage is very smooth and slippery. It provides a cushion between the bones and allows the bones to have a smooth gliding action. When the cartilage begins to break down due to overuse, high-impact activities such as running and jumping, and age, it begins to cause pain. It can be fixed by joint replacement, which is a type of treatment many people receive. Or we can help the body regrow or repair the cartilage that has been broken down. It only takes a small amount of cartilage regrowth to reduce pain. Even regrowth of about one millimeter of cartilage will influence the joint and decrease pain and reduce swelling.

Can joint damage caused by overuse, by breakdown of cartilage, by living an active life also be helped with regenerative medicine? The answer is yes, absolutely. Recently, *The Journal of Family Practice* published an article discussing prolotherapy as a non-conventional treatment for osteoarthritis. According to the study, 91% of the participants who received prolotherapy as a treatment for osteoarthritis would recommend that treatment to control their osteoarthritis.[16] Obviously, there is no guarantee for any patient or any particular condition. There is no medical procedure that can guarantee anything for that matter. If you have a physician who guarantees you an outcome, then you should perhaps consider getting a second opinion. Having said that, a number of patients who have come into my office because they suffer from osteoarthritis have been helped by prolotherapy, PRP, or stem cells.

I'd like to share the case of a 67-year-old male who came to me. He was experiencing pain in his knees, and he was unable to walk long distances without any significant pain and swelling. He was also having trouble sleeping due to the pain. I commonly see this as a source of insomnia. This patient had been told that he needed to have a knee replacement, which he was adamant that he did not want. A friend of a friend told him to contact me to discuss treatment options and see if there was anything that could be done. I distinctly remember him saying, "Doc, I'm skeptical, but I'm desperate. I'm willing to try anything." It was September when I first saw him, and he had a hunting trip planned for December, so we had a lot of work to do to take him from experiencing pain on even simple, short-distance walking to being able to go on an extended hunting trip. There was a short time—just three months—to accomplish his big goal of being able to go on this hunting trip. We had a conversation about what was going on and what my assessment was, and we decided to do an aggressive treatment course to get him ready for his hunting trip. After the first treatment, he noticed a decrease in pain. After the second treatment, he started hiking in preparation for his trip. We did a total of four or five treatments, and he was able to leave for his trip as planned. I don't

16 Slattengren, A.H., Christensen, T., Prasad, S., & Jones, K. (2014). PURLs: Prolotherapy: A nontraditional approach to knee osteoarthritis. *The Journal*

know who of us was most excited that he was able to go on this trip that he had wanted to go on for 20 years.

I get to see amazing results like this regularly, but I have never lost my excitement and amazement for the body's ability to heal, recover, and restore its function. I hope I never will lose the excitement or the feeling of amazement in watching patients regain what they once thought was lost.

---

of Family Practice, 63(4), 206–208. Retrieved December 2, 2015, from http://www.ncbi.nlm.nih.gov/pmc/articles/PMC4042896/

CHAPTER 6

I Don't Want to Have Surgery

Surgery is a wonderful tool that saves many lives every day. It is used in emergency situations, trauma, and even electively. Medical technology has made it possible for us to save lives, extend lives, provide comfort, improve our quality of life, and even enhance ourselves cosmetically. It is amazing how far we have come in the last several years. I'm very thankful for the advances that have been made in surgical procedures, and I am very grateful for skilled surgeons. Without them, I wouldn't be alive today.

However, I'm also thankful that there are alternatives to surgery, and this is where I come in. Despite all the advances in medicine, many people are still averse to having surgery. When patients come to my office, it's not uncommon for them to say that they don't want to have surgery or that they want to postpone surgery for as long as possible even if they realize that it's inevitable. Is it possible to skip surgery when your doctor tells you that it's the next step? The short answer is maybe.

Common Misdiagnoses

Before embarking on surgery to correct the problem, it is important to be sure that the problem is the problem. I have seen a number of surgeries for misdiagnosed conditions that did nothing to relieve the pain the surgery was intended to resolve.

Carpal tunnel. Carpal tunnel syndrome, also called median nerve syndrome, is estimated to cause more than three million cases of numbness and tingling in the hands— specifically the thumb, the index, the middle finger, and part of the ring finger—every year. The NIH (the National Institute of Health) describes this condition as the compression of the median nerve at the wrist. It is thought to be caused by repetitive use of the hands causing swelling or thickening of the tendon that runs through a very narrow canal in the forearm into the palmar surface of the hand called the carpal tunnel.[17]

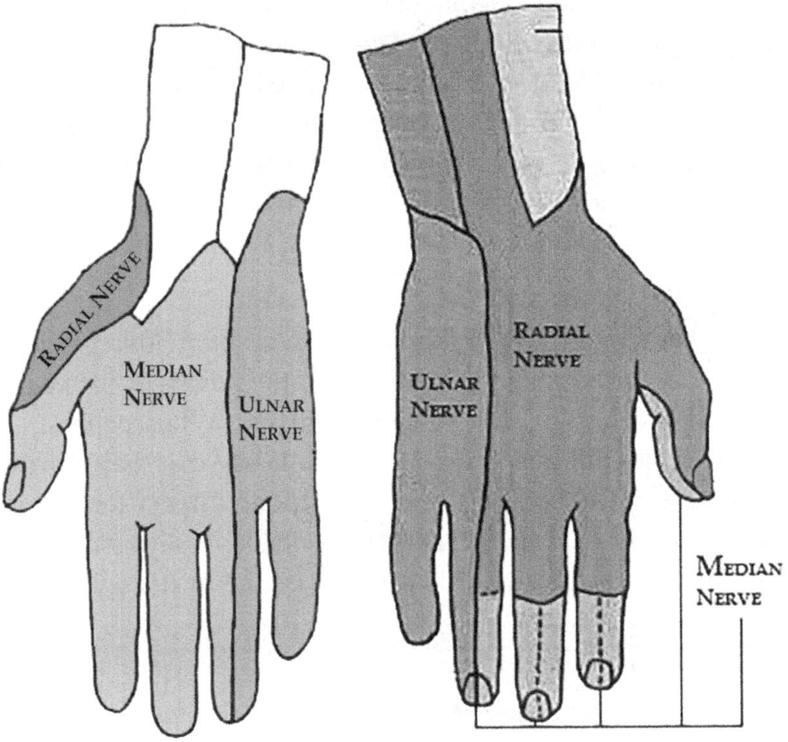

17 NIH (n.d.). *Carpal Tunnel Syndrome Fact Sheet.* Retrieved December 3, 2015, from http://www.ninds.nih.gov/disorders/carpal_tunnel/detail_carpal_tunnel.htm

There is no doubt this condition can be debilitating, but I believe carpal tunnel syndrome is often a misdiagnosis for other neuropathic (nerve) pain that is affecting the median nerve. From the region where the median nerve exits the spine in the neck to the fingers, there are multiple points that can cause nerve compression and subsequently numbness, tingling, pain, and immobility of the hands. The carpal tunnel is just one of the areas where this can occur. Don't forget about the elbow, the shoulder, damage to the cervical spine such as cervical herniation, whiplash injury, vertebral fusion (whether surgical or natural), and facet syndrome of the neck, just to name a few of the other causes of median nerve impingement.

Carpal tunnel surgery is very common, but surgery isn't the only option for treating this nerve pain. Properly assessing the point of origin of the nerve compression is paramount to success in any treatment. Most people who have pain in their hands rightfully seek advice, diagnosis, and subsequent treatment from a hand surgeon.

But what happens if the pain is not generated in the area of the carpal tunnel and you have carpal tunnel surgery? You guessed it. The pain doesn't go away. This was the case for a 57-year-old female who had numbness and tingling in her hands and fingers along with a loss of grip strength and ability to bend her middle finger. After being diagnosed with carpal tunnel syndrome, she was told that surgery was the only way to repair the damage and reduce the pain. During my evaluation with her, I ordered a nerve conduction velocity test (NCV) to assess the origin of the compression. The test revealed significant neuropathy and myopathy—nerve and muscle damage—but it wasn't necessarily related to the carpal tunnel. Considering her history of neck injury, it made sense to me to start at the root of the nerves where they exit the spine and work our way down. Due to some other health issues, we decided to start with a very non-invasive approach to begin healing the nerve. We utilized herbs, vitamins, minerals, and some amino acids, which are the building blocks of nerves, to repair her system. Within one month, she started feeling a decreased amount of pain as well as increased mobility in her fingers. Her grip strength increased, and she was able to hold large objects, which was something she hadn't been able to do before treatment. Before we started, she had difficulty doing simple things like holding a glass to take a drink of water or picking up her handbag from the ground. After several months of this treatment plan, we began using PRP injections to repair the significant damage in her neck. The multiple past injuries of the cervical spine had caused cervical instability, which we were able to repair. Sometimes pain in the hands and fingers is carpal tunnel syndrome, and sometimes it's not. An accurate diagnosis is key to an accurate treatment. If the procedure doesn't treat the problem, it will not provide a resolution, no matter how powerful it is. For this patient, surgery would have been unnecessary and ineffective, not to mention expensive.

Piriformis syndrome. Another common misdiagnosis I see is piriformis syndrome. This is a condition where a small muscle in the buttocks region spasms. The muscle is responsible for external hip rotation and is used in many activities. The spasms in this muscle can create a compression of the sciatic nerve causing pain that radiates down from the backside of the buttock all the way down the leg and as far as the foot. This pain can be similar to sciatic pain and a lot of people, including doctors, think that is what it is. Since it is caused by the piriformis muscle, it's not actually sciatica. Sciatica is due to a spinal injury whereas piriformis syndrome is a spasm of a muscle. If we were to treat the spinal injury with surgery, which is fairly common, the muscle spasm of a non-related muscle would not be resolved. Therefore, the surgery would be an ineffective and unnecessary treatment.

When we think about pain that radiates down the posterior side of the body, from the buttocks to the foot, we commonly think of sciatic nerve compression. It's a good thought; the sciatic nerve is a large nerve that is the primary source of nerve function and branching in the lower body. However, there are several structural conditions that can cause referred pain mimicking sciatic pain including quadratus lumborum myofascial pain syndrome, trigger points in the posterior pelvic floor muscles, gluteus maximus muscle, gluteus medius muscle, and gluteus minimus muscle. In addition to the muscular structures, we can't forget about the facet joints of the lumbar spine and ligament laxity in the lumbar spine, sacroiliac joint injury, or any combination of the above. Rarely does an injury happen in isolation. When the facet joints of the spine become unstable, small paraspinal muscles of the lumbar spine work to stabilize an unstable joint. In this process of protecting the spine, there can also be compression of nerves as the nerve roots exit the spinal cord at different vertebral levels called the lumbrosacral complex (L4-S3) to combine into the infamous sciatic nerve.

If an MRI rules out disc herniation causing nerve compression, the diagnosis frequently given is piriformis syndrome. In my experience, true piriformis syndrome is fairly rare. Injury to the sacroiliac joint, which subsequently causes sciatic nerve compression and pain, is far more common but often misdiagnosed as piriformis syndrome. Once the actual cause of pain is identified, the proper treatment can be administered. It increases the chance of regenerating the affected tissues, which leads to healing that results in improved function and elimination of pain.

Damages That Are Often Considered Surgical

When it comes to musculoskeletal injuries, there is a very wide range of damage that can happen. Unfortunately, many of us avoid going to the doctor when the symptoms first start. We tend to ignore them, wait, and hope for the best. But then it comes to a point when the body tells us that we can no longer ignore the symptoms. At that point, we have started looking for answers to our question. Sometimes the answer to our question is surgery, and sometimes it's not.

What happens if the pain you feel is preventing you from working? Every day is uncomfortable at best and excruciating at worst. What if you have been evaluated and told that you need surgery, for which you are not a candidate due to age or health? What happens if you can't take time off work to recover from the surgical procedure? What happens if you just don't want to have surgery? Are you then sentenced to a life of pain, of attempting to manage the pain through medication, of limited mobility, of not being able to enjoy the activities that you used to enjoy, of not being able to perform your work duties? No, not necessarily.

A 41-year-old male came to my office and presented with a torn medial meniscus. He was experiencing pain every day, and he had been told that the only thing that would help his condition was surgery. However, as a chef, he was unable to take time off for recovery from surgery. It also meant that he was on his feet for many hours each day, which aggravated his condition. He wasn't interested in medication to manage the pain, and he sincerely asked if I would give him a second opinion. After I evaluated him, I looked at his MRI. I got to know more about his medical history and understood why he was very reluctant to take any pain medication. I also took the time to understand what his medical problems were. I told him that I thought I could help him, but it would likely take more than one treatment. The relief wasn't going to be overnight, but we would start on the road to regeneration and repair of the torn meniscus. A few weeks later, I received a report from him that his knee was drastically better. He was extremely pleased with the procedure and thanked me for helping him. He was astounded by the fact that the pain in his knee was gone and that he hadn't had to miss work to recover from the procedure. I think the fact that he didn't have to spend time away from work was the best part for him. I have to admit it is very gratifying when I get this type of report.

Given what I know about regenerative medicine, is there ever a time when I think surgery is the best option? You bet. There was a 23-year-old male who came to my office with an ulnar collateral ligament injury, also known as a UCL or Tommy John injury. This patient had gotten this injury during an MMA fight. One of the first things he said to me was: "I really don't want to have surgery." He was referred to me by a former patient who had experienced good results healing his injuries. He wanted to know if there was anything I could do to help him avoid surgery. I was skeptical. I think regenerative medicine can be used for most types of injuries, but I didn't think I could help him with his Tommy John injury. First of all, this injury tends to be quite significant. Secondly, the MRI showed that the ulnar collateral ligament had sustained a complete rupture. There is not a lot that prolotherapy or PRP can do to repair a complete rupture of the ligament or tendon because, in those cases, there aren't any strands of fibers left to build upon. So in those cases, stem cells or surgery are the best options. After I had examined him and discussed the severity of his injury, I referred him to an orthopedic surgeon for evaluation. He was resistant to consult with the orthopedic surgeon because he adamantly didn't want to have surgery. During our discussion, I told him that if the surgeon felt that his injury was non-surgical, he could come back, and we would give it a shot, but there were no guarantees. Again, I was highly skeptical that regenerative medicine would work in this particular case. I had seen it repair injuries in amazing ways, but it wasn't likely that it could help a complete rupture of the ligament. Eventually, he agreed to go to the orthopedic surgeon.

A couple of weeks later, he returned because the orthopedic surgeon felt that a wait-and-see approach was best. He had begun to gain some strength in the injured area, and the orthopedic surgeon was hopeful that physical therapy would be enough to repair the injury, so he was going to undergo physical therapy while he waited. At that point, we decided to give the regenerative treatment a try, with the understanding that it was very unlikely to provide any results, especially not the result he was hoping for. Since the risk was low in my opinion, there was no harm in giving it a try at this point.

Much to my surprise, and it was a very pleasant surprise, the treatment made a significant difference in his injury. He began to heal. As a healthy athlete, the results of the treatment were quite astounding. Even I was shocked. Upon re-examination, I found myself utterly blown away by the power of the treatment and his body's ability to heal and repair itself. He was able to avoid surgery completely in a situation where I had felt that surgery was the only option.

Now, not all cases are going to end like this. There are times when, even after treatment, surgery does need to happen. Is that a failure of the therapy? I don't consider it to be that. There is nothing wrong with making the decision that surgery is the best option to heal an injury.

Osteoarthritis

When we talk about damage, damages to the ligament and tendon are very common, but these are by far not the only injuries that are considered surgical. According to the Centers for Disease Control (CDC), arthritis is the top cause of disability in the U.S., and osteoarthritis is the primary type of arthritis that causes disability. In fact, "In the United States, 23% of all adults, or about 53 million people, have arthritis. It is a leading cause of disability,"[18] and one of every two people in the U.S. population is expected to suffer from osteoarthritis by age 85.[19] While the diagnosis of osteoarthritis is predominantly in people who are 65 years and older, the CDC writes that in 2014, nearly

---

18 CDC. (2016, November 2). *Arthritis*. Retrieved February 3, 2017, from https://www.cdc.gov/chronicdisease/resources/publications/aag/arthritis.htm

19 Murphy, L., Schwartz, T. A., Helmick, C. G., Renner, J. B., Tudor, G., Koch, G., Dragomir, A., Kalsbeek, W. D., Luta, G. and Jordan, J. M. (2008), Lifetime risk of symptomatic knee osteoarthritis. *Arthritis & Rheumatism, 59* (9), 1207–1213. doi: 10.1002/art.24021

two-thirds of the reported cases of osteoarthritis were in persons younger than age 65.[20] It's not uncommon to see people in my office with osteoarthritis in their 30s and 40s.

Osteoarthritis can occur in any joint. Conventional conservative treatments are typically used first in cases of osteoarthritis. These treatments consist of the following:

- Over-the-counter pain medicines
- Analgesics and anti-inflammatory medication
- Physical therapy
- Joint realignment
- Injection therapies like cortisone or hyaluronic acid injection
- Prescription pain medication.

After what are considered to be conservative treatments have been exhausted, then joint replacement is the next option. The most commonly replaced joints are the hip joints and the knee joints. It has been reported that there are 600,000 knee replacements done each year in the U.S.[21] Obesity is cited as a contributing cause of osteoarthritis. With increasing obesity, complete knee replacement surgery (also known as arthroplasty) "is expected to exceed three million [per year] by the year 2030."[22] There is an average cost of

---

20 CDC (2015). At aA Glance 2015. *Arthritis. Addressing the Nation's Most Common Cause of Disability* [PDF file]. Retrieved February 3, 2017, from https://www.cdc.gov/chronicdisease/resources/publications/aag/pdf/2015/athritis-aag-508.pdf

21 A Nation in Motion (2017) *Beyond Surgery Day: The Full Impact of Knee Replacement.* Retrieved February 3, 2017, from http://www.anationinmotion.org/value/knee/

22 A Nation in Motion (2017) *Beyond Surgery Day: The Full Impact of Knee Replacement.* Retrieved February 3, 2017, from http://www.anationinmotion.org/value/knee/

approximately $20,000 per replacement,[23] so currently $12 billion is spent annually on knee replacements alone. Now, calculate that amount for the estimated three million replacements expected by 2030! You can't put a price on pain relief, but if you have the chance to get relief without the risk and cost associated with surgery, doesn't it make sense to explore the option?

According to some sources, 90% of knee joint replacements are considered to be successful. That means that out of 600,000 cases, there are 60,000 people who have some amount of pain post-surgery. There are a variety of reasons for this. There is not guaranteed success with surgery, and there are risks to it. Sometimes other structures become damaged inadvertently. Sometimes nerves become damaged. And sometimes there are compensatory injuries that are not addressed during the surgery. I have seen patients who have done beautifully post-surgery, but I have also seen patients who are worse off after the procedure, or series of procedures, than before. Infection, continued pain, and new nerve pain is quite common. When this happens, utilizing the body to heal itself naturally is successful, and it does address the majority of problems very well. Keep in mind that when a joint replacement is done, the pain that lingers isn't from the joint, since that is artificial. The pain comes from the supporting structures that are damaged inadvertently or were never addressed as the initial cause of the pain.

Ablation

Another common procedure is nerve ablation or neurotomy. I often see it used on people who continue to have pain after they have had a joint replacement. It is considered a non-surgical invasive injection

---

23 A Nation in Motion (2017) *Beyond Surgery Day: The Full Impact of Knee Replacement.* Retrieved February 3, 2017, from http://www.anationinmotion.org/value/knee/

and is used in an attempt to stop nerve pain. In this procedure, a radiofrequency needle is used to deliver an electrical current to the affected nerve, or the nerve that is suspected to cause the pain. This helps to isolate the nerve or nerves that register pain. Once the nerve pain is recreated by isolating the nerve that is thought to register the pain, then heat is used to heat up the nerve. This causes what is called heat lesion, which damages the nerve and interrupts the nerve's ability to send pain signals to the brain. It doesn't do anything to eliminate the pain; it just interrupts the signals so that the brain doesn't recognize that the pain is there. Nerve ablation is commonly used for spinal facet syndrome due to arthritis or spinal stenosis.

Facet syndrome can occur anywhere along the spine. It is a very common cause of back pain, leg pain, neck pain, and arm pain, and it's known as neuropathy.

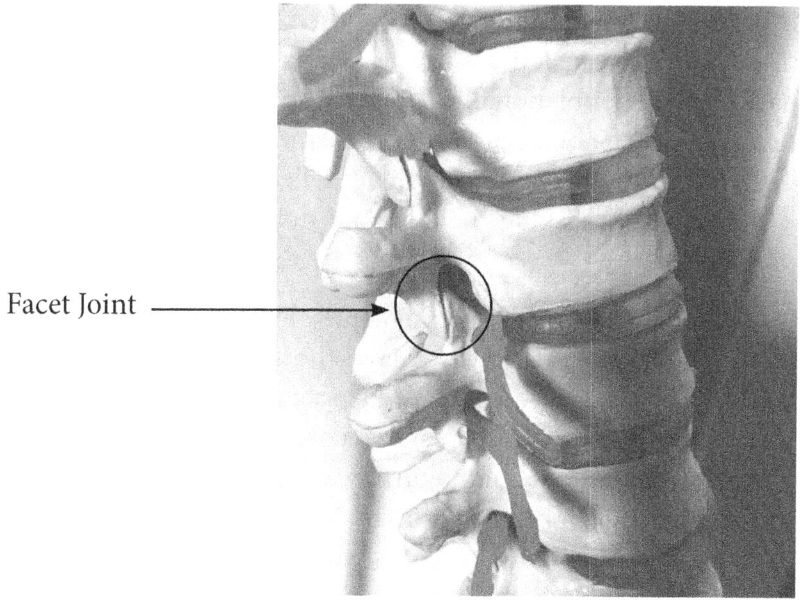

Facet joints are the joints in the spine that connect one vertebra to another. They are also sometimes called articular joints. These joints allow movement in the spine—movement bending forward and backward, movement bending side to side, and movement rotating. Nerves exit the spine along these joints, so when the joint is damaged, the possibility of nerve compression is great. Near each facet joint along the spine sit small nerves called medial nerves. If there is an underlying injury that causes instability of the spinal facet, the nerves will become compressed or aggravated as the muscles attempt to stabilize the facet joint in an effort to stabilize the spine. Facet joints also have cartilage, giving the joints a smooth, glassy surface to slide and glide on during movement. When this cartilage breaks down, it's called osteoarthritis.

In an effort to address the nerve pain caused by facet syndrome, nerve ablation can be used. The purpose of the ablation procedure is to disrupt the pain signals as opposed to correcting the issue that causes the joint instability or the facet syndrome. Once the nerves have undergone ablation, the damage is still there, and the spine is still unstable, but the brain no longer recognizes it as a painful condition. Therefore, the patient may experience relief but not healing. Now, what is the point of masking the pain and not correcting the underlying problem?

Nerve ablation isn't a permanent solution as nerve regeneration and healing occurs naturally. Even if the ablation procedure provides pain relief, the pain can be expected to return as the nerve heals, which happens within about two years. According to at least one study, the pain that is measured upon return is worse than the original pain that was treated. It is not uncommon for me to see patients come in after a nerve ablation with pain that is worse or not mediated at all after the surgery. As with any procedure, there are risks, which include infection, permanent nerve pain, and skin numbness. An additional risk is that since you no longer feel the pain, you are very likely to reinjure yourself or increase the existing injury.

Obviously, there are people who have had successful nerve ablations, knee replacements, hip replacements, and shoulder replacements. I'm not saying that medical technology never works. But for people who don't want to introduce that into the body because they are concerned about their overall health or the time it takes to recuperate from surgery or just have no desire to undergo surgery unless necessary, regenerative medicine is an amazing option. Regenerative medicine is a very promising way to repair injuries without having to turn to surgery. In some cases, surgery may be required, but it doesn't have to be the solution for every case. As I have mentioned before, I'm not against surgery, but I am against surgery when it's used as an initial course of action. I would rather try to support the body and its ability to heal naturally with the least amount of side effects possible and use surgery as a last resort. It may not prevent surgery forever; it may only postpone it, but circumstances change. Having to undergo surgery five or 10 years from now is often more tolerable to patients than having to undergo it today. Surgery can often be postponed for years.

There is nothing wrong with exploring all the options before making the decision to have a surgical repair. It is certainly not my role to dissuade anybody from having surgery, but it is my role to assess injuries accurately and give my expert opinion regarding alternatives to surgery. If I truly believe that what I have to offer can help, I will tell you that. If I believe that surgery is the best option, given all the information and circumstances, I won't hesitate to share that opinion either. I got into medicine to educate people, to talk to them about their options, and to treat them appropriately for their concerns. Will my opinion differ from another physician's? Possibly, but I have no interest in pushing procedures for the benefit of my pocketbook and the detriment of the patient.

PART II

What Your Doctor May Not Tell You

CHAPTER 7

Inflammation

One of the toughest things about being a doctor is that there seems to be an expectation that you have all the answers to every question. It's a very unrealistic expectation for patients to have for doctors and for doctors to have for themselves. Obviously, no one person is going to have all the answers. One of the things I like to discuss with my patients when they come into the office is what they may not have been told by other doctors they have been seeing. It's not to slight other doctors, but as I said, no one person can have all the answers to everything.

We have all had some injuries in our lives. The longer we live, the more likely it is we have had one or several, whether it was a twisted ankle from playing with the kids or a more significant injury from playing sports in high school, college, or professionally. When these injuries occurred, I'm sure most of us did exactly what we have been taught to do: ice it and wrap it, and then use anti-inflammatory drugs to control the swelling. That is typically how we treat injuries, regardless of whether it is a recent injury or an injury that happened several years ago. If that is the way you have treated your injuries in the past, don't worry. We all do the best we can. When we know better, then we can do better. So let's chat about a few things your doctor may not be telling you in regards to how to treat injuries.

The Inflammatory Process

Earlier, we talked about the inflammatory process. The inflammatory response is the first thing that happens when we have a tissue injury. It is accompanied by pain, swelling, heat, and loss of mobility. There is widely distributed information that inflammation is bad and that we want to shut it down at all costs. However, it's important to remember that inflammation has a protective purpose and is a response to pathogens, infection, and tissue damage.

When we use the general term *inflammation*, what we are really talking about is the inflammatory pathway, the biochemical pathway in the body that is utilized for healing. COX, an acronym for cyclooxygenase, is an enzyme, or set of enzymes found in the inflammatory pathway. We will talk about Cyclooxygenase 1 (COX-1) and Cyclooxygenase 2 (COX-2). The COX-1 isoenzyme is involved in gastrointestinal function (digestion and elimination of food), whereas COX-2 is inflammatory and produces prostaglandins. Prostaglandins are the chemicals that will kick off regeneration and healing of the tissue or injury. They are responsible for promoting inflammation, pain, and fever.

The healing process is a fairly intricate process that is composed of three phases. The first stage is the inflammation itself, which lasts about 24 to 72 hours. The second stage is proliferation, or regrowth, which happens for about 21 days. Then, the third stage, the remodeling portion of the process, goes on for about seven days. The body is trying to repair the injury for anywhere between 21 and 28 days after it happened.

NSAIDs' Effect on the Process

It is very common to use ibuprofen or another type of nonsteroidal anti-inflammatory drug (NSAID) to treat inflammation. NSAIDs are said to be "among the most widely used medication in the world because of their demonstrated efficacy in reducing pain and inflammation."[24] It's almost second nature for many doctors to recommend the use of it. It doesn't require a prescription, although there are prescription versions of it, and many people keep it in their medicine chest at home, so it's easily accessible.

The problem with any NSAID is that it acts on the inflammation phase of the inflammatory pathway as a whole to shut it down and block inflammation, so it may make your injury worse, especially in the initial stages. NSAIDs are known as COX inhibitors. They shut down the COX enzymes that cause inflammation and release prostaglandins, which signal growth factors to the area. Subsequently, they keep us from going through the other stages. The first stages of the inflammatory process set us up for healing. If we shut down inflammation within the first phase, within the first 24 to 72 hours, then we won't get into the subsequent sections of the healing pathway where regrowth and proliferation happens.

Let's break this down a bit. Please hang in there as I get just a bit technical to explain the process.

---

24 Ong, C.K.S., Lirk, P., Tan, C.H., & Seymour, R.A. (2007). An Evidence-Based Update on Nonsteroidal Anti-Inflammatory Drugs. *Clinical Medicine and Research*, 5(1),19-34. doi:10.3121/cmr.2007.698.

Inflammatory Pathway

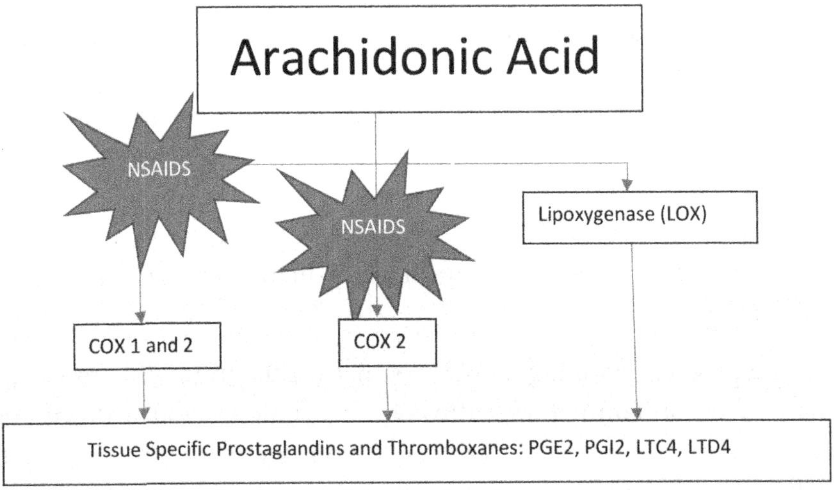

Ibuprofen and other anti-inflammatory medications affect the two enzymes COX-1 and COX-2. NSAIDs come in both nonselective and selective COX inhibitors. The nonselective COX inhibitors block the COX enzymes as a whole. It's also where we get the concern of gastrointestinal effects such as heartburn and ulcer. Ibuprofen, diclofenac, and naproxen are examples of non-selective COX inhibitors. Selective COX inhibitors target either the COX-1 or the COX-2 enzymes. These selective, specific COX-2 inhibitors, such as Celebrex, are often used to circumvent the gastrointestinal problems caused by using ibuprofen or other non-selective COX inhibitors. COX-2 inhibitors were once considered inferior in analgesic (pain relief) action, but recent comparisons of COX-2 NSAIDs to non-specific NSAIDs show that the analgesic effect is comparable.[25] However, there has been a recent concern of cardiovascular effect of using COX-2 specific inhibitors.

---

25 Ong, C.K.S., Lirk, P., Tan, C.H., & Seymour, R.A. (2007). An Evidence-Based Update on Nonsteroidal Anti-Inflammatory Drugs. *Clinical Medicine and Research,* 5(1),19-34. doi:10.3121/cmr.2007.698.

It stands to reason that if the gastrointestinal effects of a non-specific NSAID are associated with inhibiting the COX-1 enzyme, then it should be safer to use a COX-2 inhibitor. The problems that have been reported in recent literature, however, dispute that thought. Inhibiting only the COX-2 enzyme creates an imbalance, which could lead to arterial wall damage or arterial clotting. That could lead to a fatal event such as a myocardial infarction (heart attack), pulmonary embolism (blood clot in the lung), or stroke.

When the COX enzymes are affected, we get a complete shutdown of that entire inflammatory pathway. When that inflammation is blocked, the pain does decrease, which is what most people want. But don't forget that pain is a part of the natural healing process. Why would we want to shut down the natural healing process?

According to *Sports Medicine Journal:*

> Arguably the most important of these processes is inflammation since it is a consistent and lasting response. The inflammatory response is dependent on two factors, namely the extent of actual physical damage and the degree of muscular vascularization at the time of injury. However, long-term anti-inflammatory treatment is not necessarily effective in promoting healing, as indicated by various studies on NSAID treatment.[26]

The authors of this article recognize the effect of using NSAIDs at the time of acute injuries and what happens when we use them to treat chronic injuries.

---

[26] Smith, C., Kruger, M.J., Smith, R.M., & Myburgh, K.H. (2008). The inflammatory response to skeletal muscle injury: illuminating complexities. *Sports Medicine Journal. 38*(11), 947-69. doi: 10.2165/00007256-200838110-00005

Other Effects of NSAIDs

Some time ago, it was decided that, in medicine, we would look at the body as systems. We would look at the cardiovascular system as an entity in and of itself. We would look at the endocrine system as an entity in and of itself. We would look at the musculoskeletal system as an entity in and of itself. It was somehow forgotten that all the interactions of each one of those systems make up the body as a whole. These systems don't work in a vacuum; they are interconnected. When we assess one area, it's likely that we are assessing one or many other areas in the body.

NSAIDs have many additional effects on the body. It's important to note that studies discuss the vast adverse effect of using NSAIDs:

> NSAIDs are associated with a number of adverse effects. These include alterations in renal function, effects on blood pressure, hepatic injury and platelet inhibition which may result in increased bleeding.[27]

Let's take a moment to discuss the effect of platelet inhibition. PRP treatment relies directly on the chemical signaling of inflammation created by the platelets as they are directed to the injury via the immune response, so inhibiting platelets will render the treatment ineffective. Prolotherapy and stem cell treatments are affected in the same manner. By inhibiting the body's natural ability to heal, injuries progress from acute to chronic.

NSAIDs increase bleeding, which leads to increased mucosal damage (damage to mucosal cells in the body, cells that create mucus). Mucosal damage can happen any place that is slippery in the body,

---

27 Ong, C.K.S., Lirk, P., Tan, C.H., & Seymour, R.A. (2007). An Evidence-Based Update on Nonsteroidal Anti-Inflammatory Drugs. *Clinical Medicine and Research,* 5(1),19-34. doi:10.3121/cmr.2007.698.

from the nose to the eyeballs to the stomach to the intestines. All those areas are mucosal lined. Mucosal damage can result in ulcers and intestinal permeability.

NSAIDs also decrease the blood flow to the stomach. When that happens, it decreases the digestion of food. A decreased digestion of food increases the chance of being nutrient depleted and creating what is called intestinal permeability, which can result in food sensitivity.

Taking NSAIDs on a consistent basis can also lead to a decreased blood flow to the kidneys. This is called renal profusion, and it directly increases blood pressure. It also leads to a higher risk of cardiovascular disease and stroke.

Another consequence of taking NSAIDs is that it decreases the amount of glutathione in the body. Glutathione is the master antioxidant, which plays a role in the liver. It detoxifies medications, pesticides, solvents, and all the things that we are exposed to by eating, breathing, or drinking. It's also related to cardiovascular and cancer protection. It's instrumental in producing energy in the cell's mitochondria, also known as the powerhouse of the cell, so decreased glutathione can have an effect on our energy level.

The NSAIDs like aspirin and ibuprofen decrease the ability to metabolize hormones, such as estrogen and thyroid hormones, properly because they slow down an enzyme in the cyclooxygenase pathway. This can lead to migraines, mood disorders, thyroid imbalances, and other hormone imbalances.

Any use of any type of anti-inflammatory or even pain-relieving medicine, such as acetaminophen, can have far-reaching effects. A recent study in *Science Daily* talked about how NSAIDs will decrease fertility after just 10 days of use. Although most non-prescription pain relievers do not result in severe effects in healthy people, some of the most commonly used NSAIDs have potentially deadly side effects. These NSAIDs include aspirin and drugs containing ibuprofen, such as naproxen, Advil, and Aleve. "Researchers say 16,500 people die and 103,000 people are hospitalized each year because of NSAID-related problems."[28] We come back to the issue of using a drug to mask or suppress pain as opposed to fixing pain, and the long-term effects of using that strategy.

The point of this conversation is to help you understand the far-reaching effects of anti-inflammatory medication. Not only do they increase the chances of chronic injury, but they also pose all these other risks like ulcers, high blood pressure, decreased fertility, loss of energy, and hormonal disorder. As you can see, there are dangers to using NSAIDs that, in my opinion, outweigh the benefits of decreasing pain, especially when there are other options for pain control. It's paramount not to use NSAIDs as a primary means of controlling pain, specifically on a chronic, ongoing basis. Many people take them at too high a dosage, and they end up with severe effects.

Ice and Its Effect on Injury

One of the essential elements of the healing process of a tissue injury is circulation to the area. When circulation increases, blood flow increases, causing increased nutrients to the area and increased waste removal. As I said earlier, when inflammation happens, it causes pain, swelling, and heat. All those things occur because blood and lymph, which flows right along with the blood vessels, move into that area and create a circulatory effect.

When we put ice on the injured area, we constrict those vessels, constricting blood flow, especially when we apply ice for long periods of time. Some doctors promote applying ice 15 to 20 minutes at a time,

---

28 WebMD (2003, January 30). *When Relieving the Pain Raises the Risk.* Retrieved February 3, 2017, from http://www.webmd.com/pain-management/news/20030130/when-relieving-pain-raises-risk#1

and most people do that several times a day because it helps decrease the pain associated with inflammation, so it provides comfort. Like NSAIDs, ice shuts down or slows down circulation to the injured area.[29] As a result, we decrease the number of nutrients coming into the area and the amount of waste being removed. Fewer nutrients and less waste flow in and out of the area leading to decreased healing.

There have been several additional studies that have looked into the use of ice as a treatment and the effects on post workout recovery. The *European Journal of Applied Physiology* published a study on how using cold pack applications lead to long-term injuries in sprinters.[30] In this study, they looked at people who were running track competitively to figure out whether their use of cold packs post activity was enhancing or hurting their ability to recover. What they found from the study was that it hurt their ability to recover.

As opposed to muscles, tendons and ligaments are avascular, meaning they have no blood vessels. For that reason, they are at a disadvantage when it comes to healing. In a ligament or tendon, nutrients and waste get exchanged through diffusion. That means nutrients have to be diffused into the area as opposed to being directly delivered by a vessel. We heal much faster from a bone break than a ligament or a tendon injury, strain, or tear because there is a lot of blood flow in bones, just like in muscles. When we put ice on an

---

29 Nemet, D., Meckel, Y., Bar-Sela, S., Zaldivar, F., Cooper, D. M., & Eliakim, A. (2009). Effect of local cold-pack application on systemic anabolic and inflammatory response to sprint-interval training: a prospective comparative trial. *European Journal of Applied Physiology*, 107(4), 411–417. doi:10.1007/s00421-009-1138-y

30 Nemet, D., Meckel, Y., Bar-Sela, S., Zaldivar, F., Cooper, D. M., & Eliakim, A. (2009). Effect of local cold-pack application on systemic anabolic and inflammatory response to sprint-interval training: a prospective comparative trial. *European Journal of Applied Physiology, 107*(4), 411–417. doi:10.1007/s00421-009-1138-y

injured ligament or tendon, we make it even more difficult for the body to heal itself because we shut down an already slow process.

Hydrotherapy

If the injured area swells up like a big balloon, we want to control and bring down the swelling and modulate the amount of pain. What I would contend is a better source of treatment, rather than simply placing ice on the injured area, is to use a type of hydrotherapy. *Hydrotherapy* is just a fancy word for the use of water, specifically using differing temperatures to create an effect. Using alternating hot and cold hydrotherapy, we use hot and cold water to create increased circulation and therefore speed healing. Think about this with me: The fastest way to move any fluid—whether it is brake fluid in your brake lines or water in your garden hose—is to install a pump. That is, in a way, what we do with hydrotherapy: We install a pump. When we apply alternating temperatures of hot and cold onto the area, we make the vessels contract and dilate. When we use a cold temperature on the skin, the vessels contract. When we use a hot temperature on the skin, the vessels dilate. As this is happening, the effect on the vessels at the surface of the skin will cause the vessels deeper in the body to do the opposite action. For example, when we put heat on the surface, the surface vessels will dilate while the deeper vessels will constrict. When we alternate putting cold on the surface, the vessels on the surface will constrict, and the deeper vessels will dilate. We do this in an alternating fashion, which causes the vessels to get small and then big, and then small, and then big, and so on, thus creating a pump. The effect is increased circulation and healing of the injury. This allows us to get all the growth factors and healing chemicals we need to the area and facilitate faster and long-lasting healing.

The treatment would consist of three to five minutes of hot and 30 seconds of cold, repeating three times and always ending on cold.

The exact temperature of the treatment isn't relevant, but here are some guidelines to help. For the hot portion of the treatment, you want the water or heat source to be hot enough to turn your skin pink, but not hot enough to scald you. An ice pack or iced towel is a great way to get the flash of cold needed. If you have a break in the skin or compromised circulation due to disease or injury, this treatment would not be a good treatment for you to use, as the risk of injury is high. Please consult your naturopathic physician to ensure the safety of this treatment in your condition.

Whenever a patient, family member, or friend has an injury, after assessment, I suggest that they forego an ice-only treatment and replace it with an alternating hot and cold treatment. The latter will support and facilitate the natural healing process of the body and give the best chance of healing the injury without additional medical intervention.

Cortisone

In my office, I am often asked about the use of cortisone versus prolotherapy or PRP. Cortisone shots are very common. It's a treatment that is used for pain and inflammation. Why use cortisone to address pain and inflammation? The short answer is because it works—sometimes. Many people experience pain relief from cortisone shots, at least temporarily.

On the flip side, many people report that cortisone shots have little to no effect, especially when getting more than one shot. Why is this? Cortisone is a steroid. Its purpose is to act as an anti-inflammatory agent—to decrease inflammation and the pain associated with it. But cortisone does nothing to heal the injury. On the contrary, I would argue that cortisone shots set you up for long-term injury much in the same way that long-term use of anti-inflammatory medications, such as ibuprofen, do. You can only get two to three cortisone injections before you start destroying the joints. Not to mention the effects that cortisone can have in other areas of the body, including the adrenal glands and pancreas. The purpose of healing a long-term injury is to heal the joints and the damage. The purpose is not to suppress or mask the damage. Cortisone both suppresses and masks, but it does nothing to heal.

Many orthopedic sports medicine and "conventional" journals recognize that regenerative medicine is the way to heal the body instead of masking and suppressing the symptoms. The *Journal of Orthopedic Science* recently published a study where they compared cortisone shots to prolotherapy. They found that prolotherapy provided more long-term benefit and pain reduction than corticosteroid injections.[31] In a study published by *Foot & Ankle International*, they looked at PRP in relation to corticosteroid injection treatment in the case of severe plantar fasciitis. Plantar fasciitis is often a misdiagnosis. In true plantar fasciitis, cortisol steroid injections are common to reduce inflammation, and therefore, alleviate pain. In this study regarding plantar fasciitis, PRP was found to be more effective than corticosteroid treatments.[32]

In my experience, when people have an injury but don't feel the pain, they do silly things. If they have an injured area, and they receive something that completely shuts down the pain, they are not going to feel any feedback from the body that says, "Hey, maybe you shouldn't be doing this." Then they will just go ahead and do it, thus creating a worse injury. For example, many athletes receive cortisone shots before their performances. The shots will take away their pain, and

---

31 Jahangiri, A., Moghaddam, F.R., & Najafi, S. (2014). Hypertonic dextrose versus corticosteroid local injection for the treatment of osteoarthritis in the first carpometacarpal joint: a double-blind, randomized clinical trial. *Journal of Orthopedic Science,* 19(5), 737-743. doi: 10.1007/s00776-014-0587-2

32 Monto, R.R. (2014). Platelet-rich plasma efficacy versus corticosteroid injection treatment for chronic severe plantar fasciitis. *Foot & Ankle International, 35*(4), 313-8. doi: 10.1177/1071100713519778.

then they will perform on their injured ankle, knee, shoulder, you name it, making the injury worse.

The body is made to be in balance, so for every action, there is a counteraction. The inflammation process is very much the same.

CHAPTER 8
Other Factors That Affect Injuries and Healing

Movement

Lifestyle has become a big buzzword, especially when we talk about health. I'm not a particular fan of buzzwords. However, I will say that there are aspects of the American lifestyle that are contributing to injuries. We talk about how being sedentary contributes to obesity, but we don't talk about how it may be contributing to musculoskeletal injuries.

Current statistics on back injury are staggering. The number of people who are affected by low back pain is astronomical. We do less physical labor in today's society than we did at any other time in our history. My grandfather, who was both a farmer and a uranium miner, didn't complain about back pain and didn't have ways to evaluate back pain. He just worked through the pain. At the same time, as I remember, he never missed a chance to complain about anything. If his back had been hurting, we would have all known about it. So what is different?

Before getting into medicine, I worked in information technology. I had several roles over the course of my career, but the one thing that these roles had in common was sitting. I would sit for long periods of time. I fell prey to the work-through-lunch mentality. I was often the first one to the office and the last one to leave. I worked anywhere from 80 to 100 hours a week, and I probably spent 95% of that time sitting. What does this have to do with injury? After all, unless I fell out of my chair, sitting would be quite safe, wouldn't it? Well, no. It's not safe at all. In fact, we know that being sedentary is a huge contributing factor to injury. If we are unable or unwilling to move, we are more susceptible, directly and indirectly, to musculoskeletal injury, according to *Biomechanics of Musculoskeletal Injury.*[33]

The chances are that your doctor has recommended that you exercise a few times a week, especially if you are overweight. But when was the last time your doctor told you to get up and move to prevent an injury, or better yet, to treat an injury? Often, when my patients ask me, "How long do I need to stay off my ankle?" I tell them, "Quite frankly, I don't want you staying off your ankle. I want you moving. I want you to be smart about your moving. I don't want you to begin running on an injured ankle or knee. I don't want you to go to the gym and start lifting heavy weights with an injured shoulder or elbow, but I want you moving. I want the circulatory effects that exercise brings. So go for a walk. Walk around the block. Take the dog for a walk. Go to the park and play with your kids. Take a swim. Be smart. Do what you feel like you are up to, and listen to your body, but get up and move."

When we talk about healing forces, we can also pull in some physics. With the type of treatments I do with regenerative medicine, I want people moving. I want those joints working in a normal fashion. For example, if you have an injury in your knee, I want you to get up and walk. I don't want you immobilized. I don't want to put you in a brace. I don't want the knee wrapped. I don't want it in a cast. I

---

33 Whiting, W.C., & Zernicke, R.F. (2008). Biomechanics of MusculoskelatalMusculoskeletal Injury (2nd ed., pp. 54). Champaignng, IL: Human Kinetics Publishers.

don't want you on crutches. I want you to use that joint as you would normally use it. It's not uncommon for me to recommend for people to ride a stationary bike, walk on a treadmill, walk around the block, or go for a swim within 24 hours of having an injury or treatment with regenerative medicine. That way, they get their heart rate up and their circulation going, which is always good for healing. Especially in the use of PRP and stem cell therapy, the friction that occurs in the joint during normal use signals the stem cells to proliferate and regrow faster. We want to utilize the vector forces to create the pressure needed because the cells will respond better when they are being used. Cartilage cells regenerate better when they have pressure and the joint is used normally. It's about being smart about your usage while getting up and moving to heal as well as prevent injury.

Hormones

Another thing your doctor may not be discussing with you, especially in regards to musculoskeletal injury, is hormones. In my experience, many doctors, except endocrinologists, pay little to no attention to their patients' hormonal balance.

We all have a very small view of the number of hormones that keep us going every day. Most people think of hormones as the three chemicals estrogen, progesterone, and testosterone. If you ask a husband what hormones are, he may say that they are the chemicals that turn his beautiful and loving wife into an unpredictable pile of mush, seemingly without warning. But let's not pick on the women here. It's true that women have different hormone fluctuations than men, but we all have the same number of hormones overall, albeit hormone levels vary between genders. You may be surprised to know that there are over 70 hormones flowing through your body at any given time!

You might be asking yourself: How do my hormones relate to my tendons? Hormones are the chemical messengers that go from one part of the body, a gland, to a cell in some other part of the body to tell that cell what it's supposed to do. Some hormones are directly involved in healing and regeneration. So if hormones are not functioning properly, the body doesn't have the right messages going to the right cells to promote healing of any type, in our case musculoskeletal healing. When a patient isn't responding to treatment the way I expect, it can very well come down to a hormonal imbalance. Let's take testosterone for example. Testosterone is an anabolic steroid, which means it builds things. When testosterone is imbalanced, healing is affected in both men and women.

The hormones I see most commonly out of balance are sex hormones including estrogen, progesterone, testosterone; adrenal hormones like cortisol; thyroid hormones; and vitamin D. When vitamin D was discovered, it was misnamed. They thought it was a vitamin, but later on, they realized it was a hormone. When we fix the imbalance of hormones, the injury begins to heal. It comes down to the simple concept of giving the body what it needs to function and getting out of the way.

Antibiotics

Probably all of us have had some infection at some point. What do infections have to do with musculoskeletal injuries? Remember, I mentioned that the body doesn't work in a vacuum. In a society where we use antibiotics as an answer to all, we may be causing significant damage to connective tissue and nerves without realizing it.

One commonly prescribed antibiotic is called Fluoroquinolone. You probably would know it more commonly by Cipro or ciprofloxacin. Your doctor may not tell you that using this very common antibiotic can be a cause at worst, and a contributing factor at best, of tendon injury.

In fact, the FDA has issued a black-box warning on Cipro for Achilles tendon ruptures because we commonly see the Achilles tendon as the most affected tendon injury caused by Fluoroquinolone. But it is not the only tendon that can be affected by far. Fluoroquinolone has also been linked to hormone dysfunction and mood imbalances, as it is an inhibitor of sulfurtransferase enzymes in the liver. These are the same enzymes that are affected by acetaminophen, ibuprofen, and Aspirin. These particular enzymes in the liver are responsible for helping us metabolize hormones including sex hormones like estrogen, thyroid hormones, dopamine, and epinephrine.

As you can see, the simple use of an antibiotic, especially on a long-term basis or at very high dosages, may cause hormone imbalances. This imbalance inhibits healing of musculoskeletal injuries in an efficient manner. I have also seen some cases where antibiotics have caused connective tissue damage and nerve tissue damage, and they have been known to cause cardiovascular damage.

Judicious use of antibiotics is always the way to go. I'm not against antibiotics by any means. They have their place, and they are great advances in medicine. However, using them for every sniffle, ache, and pain doesn't make sense. It would be like shooting a mosquito with a cannon. There are ways to alleviate an infection without creating a risk of tendon rupture. Make sure that if your doctor prescribes a Fluoroquinolone, you discuss it with her or him. Are there other options for your particular condition? What is your risk of having a musculoskeletal injury caused by Fluoroquinolone toxicity, or even a single use of Fluoroquinolone? There have been studies that have linked Fluoroquinolone toxicity to patients who suffer from low back pain.[34]

---

[34] Strauchman, M., & Morningstar, M. W. (2012). Fluoroquinolone toxicity symptoms in a patient presenting with low back pain. *Clinics and Practice, 2*(4), e87. doi:10.4081/cp.2012.e87

Narcotic Pain Medication

In our conventional medical system, there seem to be very few answers to dealing with pain. Our options seem limited to pain medication (over the counter and prescriptions), cortisone shots, other steroids, and surgery. Many patients with reoccurring or chronic pain use narcotic pain medication as a way to manage the pain.

Pain medication is beneficial when used properly, but in our society, we have an unfortunate tendency to overuse things. The use of prescription medications has significantly skyrocketed. From 1999 to 2008, there was reported a 300% increase.[35] I would argue that from 2008 to current date, it has probably increased by at least another 50%. We think that if a little will do a little good, a lot will do a lot of good. With this medication, that is not the way it goes. When we think about drugs, we don't think about narcotic medications prescribed by doctors. We think about cocaine, heroin, or meth. But there are more fatal overdoses of prescription medications for pain management than there are of what we consider street drugs. The CDC reports that the number of fatal overdoses of prescription medication is higher than overdoses of cocaine and heroin combined. In 2008, the CDC reported "nearly 36,000 people dying of fatal overdoses of prescription drugs."[36] "Nearly three in every four prescription drug overdoses are being caused by prescription painkillers."[37] "We see a precedent arise

---

35 CDC. (2011, November 4). *Vital signs: Overdoses of Pprescription Opioid Ppain Relievers — United States, 1999-2008.* Retrieved February 3, 2017, from https://www.cdc.gov/mmwr/preview/mmwrhtml/mm6043a4.htm?s_cid=mm6043a4_w

36 CDC. (2011, November 4). *Vital signs: Overdoses of Pprescription Opioid painPain Relievers — United States, 1999-2008.* Retrieved February 3, 2017, from https://www.cdc.gov/mmwr/preview/mmwrhtml/mm6043a4.htm?s_cid=mm6043a4_w

37 CDC. (2011, November 4). *Vital signs: Overdoses of Pprescription Opioid Ppain Relievers — United States, 1999-2008.* Retrieved February 3, 2017, from https://www.cdc.gov/mmwr/preview/mmwrhtml/mm6043a4.htm?s_cid=mm6043a4_w

in overdose death in the US. Many Americans may be playing a very dangerous game of Russian Roulette."[38]

You will inevitably have an injury at some point. You may have had some as a kid. You may have some as an adult. You may not be a very active adult, which is going to lead to more effects of injury and pain. You may also be a very active adult, which may cause you to wear out your joints. There is no way around it. Pain is a great motivator. People will do astronomical things to get themselves out of pain. What I would propose to you is that you look into treatments that address the cause of the pain as opposed to using a NSAID or an opioid (narcotic medication) as an ongoing pain management strategy. Is the pain caused by a ligament or tendon tear? Is it caused by a herniated disk? What is the cause? Let's treat that. These are some of the things that your doctor may not be discussing with you. Feel free to bring them up. Find out how your doctor feels about them. She or he may very well have a different opinion. As I said, no one of us knows everything. No one has the answer to every question.

---

[38] CDC. (2011, November 4). *Vital signs: Overdoses of Pprescription Opioid painPain Relievers — United States, 1999-2008.* Retrieved February 3, 2017, from https://www.cdc.gov/mmwr/preview/mmwrhtml/mm6043a4.htm?s_cid=mm6043a4_w

CHAPTER 9

Happy 40th Birthday!

Life can be challenging. It's unpredictable, exasperating, and, at times, exhausting. It's also amazing, full of potential, and utterly unbelievable. Perspective and attitude have a lot to do with our experiences in life.

I recently asked a very diverse group of friends, colleagues, and acquaintances the following question: For those of you who are 40 years old and over, what has been the most challenging thing about being 40 plus? I was amused, shocked, and saddened by some of the answers I received. One friend noted that her biggest challenge was being diagnosed with triple negative breast cancer. Another stated that she had had two surgeries this year at 44, with no history of surgeries in her life. One of my friends posted a sign with warnings for using a go-cart. Among the listed cautions was "Do not use this equipment if you are over 40 years of age." I thought to myself, "Are you serious? Being 40 has now become a warning?"

I guess I can't be too surprised. In the office, I commonly hear complaints about metabolism, fitness results, and joint pain, which many people associate with being 40 years old. It seems like the age 40 is a magic number. Many people feel like the body begins to betray them once they turn 40. Weight can be difficult to lose, joints can get achy, and activities that used to be simple now feel more challenging. A few years ago, I was doing rotations with a senior doctor, and I heard a woman say to me, "Honey, just wait until you turn 40. The bottom falls out." I couldn't help but giggle under my breath, especially since she was younger than me.

The Ever-Changing Body

As you age, your body changes, and it can feel like it is betraying you. Remember the first time you felt this betrayal? It was probably around age 14 or so. Your voice may have been squeaky, your feet could have been stumbling blocks, or perhaps even your head felt too big for your body. It was difficult to manage all the growing pieces. If you were anything like me, you felt like there was an alien transforming in front of your eyes. You had to learn what to do with this new body—how to manage it, dress it, and hopefully love it. You then spent the next several years getting to know the new grown-up body that had morphed seemingly overnight. By the time you reach age 40, you have gotten used to navigating the world in the body you inhabit. Mentally, emotionally, and physically, you are mostly aware of your talents and limitations.

The amazing thing about life, and that includes your body, is that it's adaptable and ever changing. It's not uncommon to start noticing changes in your body, mind, and physical limits somewhere around the middle of your life, though not everyone goes through this change at the same time in life. These changes can be similar to, although not quite as drastic as, the changes you experienced during puberty. Most people have forgotten what an amazing transformation happened during the earlier stages of life. Yet here you are. You have had a big celebration. You have hit the big 4-0, and now you find yourself ready to tackle the next 40-something years of your life. But something seems very different. You find yourself walking into a room and can't remember what you went in for. You had a night out with friends, and whoa, you realized that you just aren't as young as you used to be. Getting out of bed, you feel stiff, creaky, and achy. My good friend stated it best: "I noticed a change in my metabolism, I don't recover as quickly fitness-wise, and I don't give a flip what people think about me anymore, which really isn't a challenge but more like a bonus." What the heck happened?

Since some people seem to navigate this change with little to no problem, what is it that makes the difference? It's hard to say for sure. Genetics, lifestyles, attitudes–I'm sure they all have something to do with it. The good news is you can work with your body, especially your achy joints. There are numerous reasons for achy joints from food sensitivities to environmental toxicities to hormone imbalance. Hormone imbalance could also be impeding your ability to recover faster or heal injuries properly. Your hormones will change throughout your life, so keep in mind that there are ways to manage these changes so that the influence feels less destructive. There are natural ways to work with your body so that you can continue to live a life filled with activity, joy, and adventure.

Let's talk about metabolic changes. Remember when you were 20 something, and you were eating pizza at 2:00 in the morning more times a week than not? Skinny jeans? All your jeans were skinny jeans. You didn't put much thought into making smart food choices because you felt fine and healthy, and who had time to cook anyway? Not to get into too much detail here, but I would argue that the choices you made in your younger years have contributed to how you feel today.

The good news is it's never too late to start over, to make new choices, and to be conscious of what you do to and for your body. Eating a good variety of foods that support health goes a long way to making sure that you have a healthy metabolism and joints. Focusing on whole foods versus processed foods, limiting sugar, and identifying and eliminating foods that your body is reacting negatively to will reduce aches, pains, bloating, and a myriad of other symptoms.

If you have reached the point of significant injury, joint damage, or ongoing pain conditions, your food choices will affect your ability to recover. There are foods that are proven to support joint repair, cartilage regeneration, and connected tissue regrowth. In regards to regenerative medicine, your results will be better if your hormones are balanced, if your food choices support healing, and if your digestive system allows proper nutrient absorption.

Most of us know that we need to eat more vegetables and fruits, drink more water, and limit our sugar intake. Knowing and doing are two different things. Don't underestimate the power of food in the healing process. As Hippocrates, the father of medicine stated, "Let food be thy medicine and medicine be thy food."[39]

The other thing that happens is that those of us who were active in our younger years and are active now reap the rewards in the form of achy joints, cartilage degeneration, sprains, strains, and potential joint replacements. From football to track to gymnastics, there are numerous ways we put the body through quite a beating. It was great. It was fun. It was healthy. But now the glory days have turned into the achy days. I have lived an active life as a competitive gymnast, softball player, cheerleader, tennis player, and racquetball player. I have done weight training. I'm a marathoner, CrossFitter, yogi, and obstacle course racer. I have had my share of injuries. Whiplash injuries, strains, sprains, multiple tears, and broken bones; I have had them all. I had knee surgery at the age of 14. I speak not only as a practitioner using regenerative medicine to help other people but also as an athlete who uses it to repair old injuries and new injuries alike.

As you may have noticed, I am passionate about regenerative medicine. I am passionate about the options it restores and the amazing

---

39 Hippocrates. (2017). Hippocrates quotes (author of Hippocratic writings). Retrieved February 3, 2017, from https://www.goodreads.com/author/quotes/248774.Hippocrates

way it allows us to tap into the healing power of nature; the healing ability that exists in the body. This is where regenerative medicine comes in. Your body still works. It still heals. Whether you are 20 or 80, healing still occurs even if it does take a little bit longer.

If there is one thing I want you to take away from reading this book, it's that despite the fact that you will never be 20 something again (thank goodness), you don't have to live with the aches and pains associated with aging. You have the opportunity to live a life that is full of passion, adventure, activity, and joy. For those of you who have waited until you retired to do the things you love to do, it's cruel to think of injury and pain preventing you from living the life you have always wanted. While there are no guarantees in life, and certainly not with health, you do still have options to recover that which you thought might have been lost. Celebrate, take control, and make the choices that lead you toward a life you want with the freedom of not caring what other people think. Happy 40th birthday!

PART III

Appendix

Glossary

ACL: anterior cruciate ligament

Adipose cells: fat cells

Angiogenesis: the formation of vessels

Articulation: "a joint or juncture between bones or cartilages in the skeleton of a vertebrate."[40]

Autocrine: "denoting a mode of hormone action in which a hormone binds to receptors on and affects the function of the same cell that produced it."[41]

Autologous: "derived from the same individual."[42]

Biomechanics: "the mechanics of biological and especially muscular activity."[43]

Chondrocytes: cartilage cells

Congenital: "existing at or dating from birth."[44]

Connective tissue: "a tissue of mesodermal origin that consists of various cells (as fibroblasts and macrophages) and interlacing protein fibers (as of collagen) embedded in a chiefly carbohydrate

---

40 Articulation [Def. 1a]. (n.d.). *Merriam Webster Online.* Retrieved December 11, 2015, from http://www.merriam-webster.com/dictionary/articulation

41 Autocrine [Def. 1]. (n.d.). *The Free Dictionary.* Retrieved December 11, 2015, from http://medical-dictionary.thefreedictionary.com/autocrine

42 Autologous [Def. 1]. (n.d.). *Merriam Webster Online.* Retrieved December 11, 2015, from http://www.merriam-webster.com/dictionary/autologous

43 Biomechanics [Def. 1]. (n.d.). *Merriam Webster Online.* Retrieved December 11, 2015, from http://www.merriam-webster.com/dictionary/biomechanics

44 Congenital [Def. 1a]. (n.d.). *Merriam Webster Online.* Retrieved December 11, 2015, from http://www.merriam-webster.com/dictionary/congenital

ground substance, that supports, end sheathes, and binds together other tissues, and that includes loose and dense forms (as adipose tissue, tendons, ligaments, and aponeuroses) and specialized forms (as cartilage and bone."[45]

COX inhibitor: substance, usually medication, that decreases the activity of cyclooxygenase enzyme(s).

CT Scan: "CT, or CAT scans, are special X-ray tests that produce cross-sectional images of the body using X-rays and a computer. CT scans are also referred to as computerized axial tomography."[46]

Extracellular matrix: provides structural and biochemical support of surrounding cells.[47]

Facet joint: a small joint in the spine where two adjacent vertebrae fit together.

Fascia: thick band of ligaments.

Femoral head: top of the femur bone, located in the thigh, fits into the hip socket.

Fibrin matrix: protein tissue structure that allows cell adhesion, creating a structure for new cells to grow.

---

45 Connective tissue [Def. 1]. (n.d.) *Merriam Webster Online.* Retrieved December 11, 2015, from http://www.merriam-webster.com/dictionary/connective%20tissue

46 WebMD. (2017). CT Scan. Retrieved February 3, 2017, from http://www.emedicinehealth.com/ct_scan/article_em.htm

47 Frantz, C., Stewart, K. M., & Weaver, V. M. (2010). The extracellular matrix at a glance. *Journal of Cell Science, 123*(24), 4195–4200. doi:10.1242/jcs.023820

Fibrocartilage: "A variety of cartilage that contains visible type I collagen fibers; appears as a transition between tendons or ligaments or bones.[48]

Half-life: the time required for a substance or drug to lose half of its effectiveness in the body.

Hypertonic solution: a solution that has a higher osmotic pressure than blood cells.

Interleukin: "any of various cytokines of low molecular weight that are produced by lymphocytes, macrophages, and monocytes and that function especially in regulation of the immune system and especially cell-mediated immunity."[49]

Isotonic solution: a solution with the same osmotic pressure as blood cells.

Ligament: "a tough fibrous band of tissue connecting the articular extremities of bones or supporting an organ in place."[50]

Mesenchymal cells: a type of cell that is derived from the mesenchyme (middle layer) of the forming embryo. Able to develop into connective tissue, lymphatic tissue, and circulatory tissues like blood vessels.

Mesoderm: the middle layer of tissue between the endoderm and ectoderm, in embryological development.

Mitochondria: called the powerhouse of the cell, responsible for generating energy.

---

[48] Fibrocartilage [Def. 2]. (n.d.). *TheFreeDictionary.com.* Retrieved February 21, 2017, from http://medical-dictionary.thefreedictionary.com/fibrocartilage

[49] Interleukin [Def. 1]. (n.d.). *Merriam Webster Online.* Retrieved December 11, 2015, from http://www.merriam-webster.com/dictionary/interleukin

[50] Ligament [Def. 1]. (n.d.). *Merriam Webster Online.* Retrieved December 11, 2015, from http://www.merriam-webster.com/dictionary/ligaments

MRI: "Magnetic resonance imaging (MRI) is a test that uses a magnetic field and pulses of radio wave energy to make pictures of organs and structures inside the body."[51]

Mucosal Damage: damage to mucus-producing cells.

Multipotent cells: cells that "can develop into more than one cell type."[52]

Myocytes: muscle cells

Myocardial infarction: heart attack

Neuropathic pain: "neuropathic pain is caused by a malfunction of the nervous system due to an injury or illness."[53]

Nociceptive pain: "the type of pain you feel when you burn yourself, twist your ankle or stub your toe. It is a dull or sharp aching pain that ranges from mild to severe. Nociceptive pain can usually be controlled."[54]

NSAID: nonsteroidal anti-inflammatory drugs

---

51 WebMD (n.d.). *Magnetic Resonance Imaging (MRI).* Retrieved December 11, 2015, from http://www.webmd.com/a-to-z-guides/magnetic-resonance-imaging-mri

52 New York State Stem Cell Science (n.d.). *What is the difference between totipotent, pluripotent, and multipotent?* Retrieved February 3, 2017, from https://stemcell.ny.gov/faqs/what-difference-between-totipotent-pluripotent-and-multipotent

53 St. Jude Medical (2016, December 1). *Understanding Chronic Pain.* Retrieved February 3, 2017, from https://www.sjm.com/en/patients/chronic-pain/what-is-chronic-pain?clset=af584191-45c9-4201-8740-5409f4cf8bdd%3ab20716c1-c2a6-4e4c-844b-d0dd6899eb3a

54 St. Jude Medical (2016, December 1). *Understanding Chronic Pain.* Retrieved February 3, 2017, from https://www.sjm.com/en/patients/chronic-pain/what-is-chronic-pain?clset=af584191-45c9-4201-8740-5409f4cf8bdd%3ab20716c1-c2a6-4e4c-844b-d0dd6899eb3a

Opioids: class of medication that binds to opioid receptors in the brain. Used for pain relief.

Osteocytes: bone cells

Paracrine: "denoting a type of hormone function in which hormone synthesized in and released from endocrine cells binds to its receptor in nearby cells and affects their function."[55]

PCL: posterior cruciate ligament. Ligament of the knee that prevents that knee hyperflexion.

Plantar fasciitis: inflammation of the fascia on the bottom of the foot.

Proliferate: "to grow by rapid production."[56]

Pulmonary embolism: potentially fatal blockage of an artery in the lung, usually caused by a blood clot.

Tendon: "a tough cord or band of dense white fibrous connective tissue that unites a muscle with some other part (such as a bone) and transmits the force which the muscle exerts."[57]

TMJ: temporomandibular joint

Trigger point: "a localized usually tender or painful area of the body and especially of a muscle that when stimulated gives rise to pain elsewhere in the body."[58]

---

[55] Paracrine [Def. 1]. *The Free Dictionary.* Retrieved December 11, 2015, from http://medical-dictionary.thefreedictionary.com/paracrine

[56] Proliferate [Def. 1]. *Merriam Webster Online.* Retrieved December 11, 2015, from http://www.merriam-webster.com/dictionary/proliferate

[57] Tendon [Def. 1]. *Merriam Webster Online.* Retrieved December 11, 2015, from http://www.merriam-webster.com/dictionary/tendon

[58] Trigger point [Def. 1]. *Merriam Webster Online.* Retrieved December 11, 2015, from [Def. 1]. Merriam Webster Online. Retrieved December 11, 2015, from http://www.merriam-webster.com/dictionary/trigger%20point

BIOGRAPHY

Darla L. Logan, NMD, MBA

We are what we repeatedly do. Excellence, therefore is not an act, but a habit.

—Aristotle

Dr. Darla L. Logan is an accomplished Naturopathic Medical Doctor, based in Scottsdale, AZ. She is also the respected medical director and owner of CellMed Clinics. While some patients refer to her as a "healer," she prefers to identify herself as a facilitator of change. As a physician, her objective is to discover and treat the root cause of disease rather than simply applying a Band-Aid solution. In doing so, Dr. Logan helps to restore and transform the quality of life of hundreds of patients every year.

Prior to venturing into the field of medicine, Dr. Logan explored a diversified career path in information technology from application developer to project manager to public speaker. She spent 12 years in a successful career that afforded her the opportunity to work with corporations and government entities to shape their business processes, technology solutions, and employee training.

Knowing that she always wanted to give people opportunities to improve their quality of life, Dr. Logan followed her heart and decided to change careers. She graduated as a Naturopathic Medical Doctor from Southwest College of Naturopathic Medicine. She has also earned a Masters of Business Administration (Finance) from New Mexico State University and a Bachelor of Business Administration (Business Computer Systems) from New Mexico State University.

A highlight for Dr. Logan has been successfully transitioning from the world of technology to a career in medicine. She is blessed with strong problem-solving skills, which have benefitted her and her clients and patients throughout her career, both in technology and medicine. Dr. Logan considers obstacles in life to be challenges that can always be overcome with consciousness and commitment, and she encourages her patients to view their own challenges in this light.

Dr. Logan is appreciated by her patients for her genuine and relatable nature. She meets people where they are and walks with them on their wellness journey to achieve their health goals. Uniquely, Dr. Logan has the ability to connect with patients from all walks of life and explain complex concepts in an easy-to-understand manner. By forming close connections with her patients, she is able to view them in a multidimensional fashion and not simply as a list of symptoms. She approaches each of her patients with the time, energy, and absolute care they deserve. Dr. Logan genuinely listens to what her patients are saying and makes sure that she fully understands the whole picture before she moves forward. Knowing that there is no such thing as a "one-size-fits-all model," she draws upon her deep knowledge and understanding of natural therapies and modern medicine to formulate solutions. Dr. Logan offers options for treatment that many people don't realize exist.

Dr. Logan feels honored to have the opportunity to help, learn from, and influence people on a daily basis by teaching them how to improve the quality of their lives while changing the quality of their health. When she is not helping others to live well, Dr. Logan can be found taking part in CrossFit training and competitions, obstacle course races (OCRs), and traveling. Her guilty pleasure, though, is playing with her rescue dog, Luci, affectionately called Monster. Luci has taught Dr. Logan a great deal about trust, unconditional love, and the value of a lazy afternoon.

Made in United States
Orlando, FL
04 November 2026

90201211R00066